AF871987

THE ULTIMATE FPAS SJT GUIDE

300 PRACTICE QUESTIONS

OXBRIDGE SOCIETY

Previous Editions: 2020, 2019, 2018, 2021

ISBN 978-1-915091-73-4

Published by *RAR Medical Services Limited*
www.oxbridgemedicalsociety.com

THE ULTIMATE FPAS SJT GUIDE

300 PRACTICE QUESTIONS

DR. RANJNA GARG
DR. SHIVUN KHOSLA

ABOUT THE AUTHORS

Ranjna has over 25 years of clinical teaching and research experience. She is currently based at the Princess Alexandra Hospital as a Consultant Endocrinologist. She is a PACES examiner. She has taught hundreds of junior doctors and prepared them through MRCP(PACES) postgraduate examinations and job interviews, including consultant interviews. She also teaches at the University of Leicester. She has authored many articles in peer reviewed journals and edited volumes. In her spare time, she enjoys photography, making candles and runs marathons.

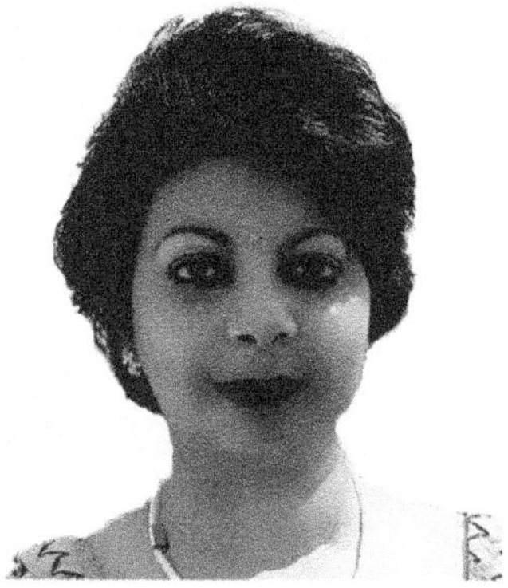

Shivun graduated from Gonville and Caius College, Cambridge with first-class honours in Biological and Biomedical Sciences before completing his clinical training in the East Anglia region, centred at Cambridge University Hospitals Trust. After spending his foundation year in Kent, Shivun is now a trainee at Guy's and St. Thomas' NHS Foundation Trust.

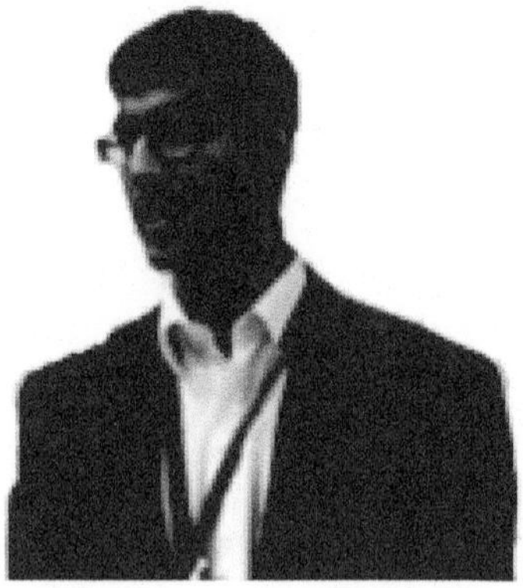

Shivun has a passion for medical education having lectured and tutored throughout his time in Cambridge to medical, veterinary, and biological science students on undergraduate and post-graduate courses. He has also implemented foundation training courses in the South Thames Foundation School, with his work being acknowledged and rewarded by Kings College London and the deanery.

Shivun achieved a total of 91.1 in his FPAS application and scored 49.1 on the SJT.

CONTENTS

INTRODUCTION

What is FPAS?

The Foundation Programme Application System (FPAS) is an online, national standardised system within the United Kingdom (UK), and is designed for final year medical students to apply for foundation training posts. It is run by the UK Foundation Programme Office (UKFPO).

What does the FPAS consist of?

FPAS consists of 10 online sections that need to be filled in so that UKFPO can ensure you have the necessary competencies to practice medicine in the UK after confirmation of passing your final examinations.

The 10 sections include:

- Personal Details
- Eligibility to practice
- Fitness to Practice
- References
- Competences
- Supplementary Evidence and Education Achievements
- Supporting Evidence (AFP only)
- Preferences for Deanery
- Equality
- Declarations

The information entered above is used to help generate a total score for your application out of a maximum of 100 points.

Section	Contributing Components	Points Available	Spread of Points
EPM	Medical School Decile Ranking	43	34-43
	Additional Degrees	5	0-5
	Publications	2	0-2
SJT	Sixty of seventy questions regarding the attributes expected of a junior doctor during their future practice	50	20-50

Why is the SJT used?

Situational Judgement Testing is a form of psychometric analysis used to assess potential employees' responses to scenarios that are frequently encountered in the workplace. It allows employers to assess aptitude for competent decision making and tests key attitudes and behaviours of potential candidates.

SJTs have been used in applications for General Practice Specialty Training for a number of years, and their success has been transitioned into the FPAS system and also the UK Clinical Aptitude Test for students applying through UCAS for A100 Medicine.

When do I sit SJT?

There are normally two sittings for the SJT – the first is normally in the first week of December; the second sitting is in the second week of January. Your medical school will decide which date you sit the exam.

Can I avoid the SJT?

Unfortunately not! Everyone applying for a foundation programme job **MUST** take the SJT. Even those who wish to apply for the Academic Foundation Programme are required to take and "pass" the SJT to fulfil the requirements set out by the UKFPO.

How is the SJT Scored?

The SJT is composed of 70 questions in a 2 hour and 20 minute exam. 10 of these questions are "plant questions." This means that they are not counted towards your final score. The total mark possible is 50.00 but virtually all students score between 20.01 and 50.00. It is worth looking at the most recent score distributions for the SJT as scores tend to cluster between 37 and 42.

SJT Points	Percentage of Applicants
0-10	0.04 %
11-20	0.14 %
21-30	1.92 %
31-35	8.82 %
36-40	35.87 %
41-45	46.66 %
46-50	6.55 %

Distribution of SJT Scores (2017)

Two-thirds of the questions are ranking questions where you receive a stem then five choices to rank in order of most appropriate to least appropriate. These are scored out of a maximum of 20 with the minimum possible mark being 8. For each answer (A-E) that is given the correct ranking (1-5), you receive 4 points. If the ranking you give is one off either way, then you receive 3 points.

For example, if you rank answer A as 2 but the examiners have it as 3, then you would receive 3 marks. If your answer is 2 ranking spots off, you receive 2 marks, if it is 3 ranking spots off, then you get 1 point. If it is 4 spots off, you receive no points. Therefore, if you make one mistake, another answer will be wrong also – thus you lose points in pairs giving an even score. For these ranking questions, you should aim for an average of 16 per question.

One-third of the questions are extended matching type questions where you will be given a choice of eight answers after a stem and will be asked to select the three best answers. Each correct answer is worth 4 marks, giving a maximum of 12 for these questions. These questions are where the majority of marks are lost as getting one option wrong loses you one-third of the available marks.

When do I get my results?

The results for the SJT are not available until March 2017 and come out on the same day as the results of your application. UKFPO do not comment on individual cases nor do they provide feedback or answer rationales.

For more information on FPAS and the SJT, we recommend reviewing the official UKFPO website.

GENERAL ADVICE

Start Early

It is much easier to prepare if you practice little and often. Start your preparation well in advance; ideally by late October to early November for the first sitting or late November for the second sitting. This way, you will have plenty of time to comfortably complete as many questions as you can, and won't have to panic just before the test, which is a much less effective and more stressful way to learn. In general, an early start will give you the opportunity to identify the complex issues and work at your own pace.

It is best to revise in a group for this type of exam. You will frequently come across questions that you do not agree with the rationales for, and therefore, getting the input of friends who have done the same question may allow you to identify different perspectives. Remember, this is what the examiners do to ultimately set the "optimal" rankings and choices, so you should do it too.

Start with the Practice Paper

Our team would recommend starting your revision with the practice paper. As this is the only official resource, doing it first gives you two advantages when coming to your revision. The first is that you get a realistic impression of the difficulty of the questions they are likely to ask and the time pressures. The second is that you can take that realism into your revision. Our editorial team know some resources are overly simple with their questions and do not reflect what you may experience as a junior doctor or in the exam.

All of our questions are based on anecdotal experiences of people from foundation to consultant level. They have been screened by an independent editorial team formed of medical students to core trainees, all of whom are experienced in medical education.

Teamwork

It is best to revise in a group for this type of exam. You will frequently come across questions that you do not agree with the rationales for, and therefore, getting the input of friends who have done the same question may allow you to identify different perspectives. Remember, this is what the examiners do to ultimately set the "optimal" rankings and choices, so you should do it too.

We would suggest creating a small revision group of four or five people and utilising the same resources so that everyone covers the same questions. Then you can sit down, discuss them together and go over rationales you felt were contentious.

THE BASICS

The Situational Judgement Test is a psychological aptitude test; it is an assessment method used to evaluate your ability for solving problems in work-related situations. SJTs are widely used in medicine as one of the criteria when deciding on applicants; it is used for the Foundation Programme and GP applications.

The aim of the SJT is to assess your ability to understand situations that you could encounter as a junior doctor and how you would deal with them. It is a method to test some of the qualities required in a healthcare professional (e.g. integrity and ability to work in a team).

The series of scenarios include possible actions and considerations. You will be asked to assess the "appropriateness" of options in relation to the scenario.

You should subdivide the options into:

- A very appropriate thing to do – This is an ideal action.
- Appropriate, but not ideal – This option can be done but is not necessarily the best thing to be done.
- Inappropriate, but not awful – This should not be done, but if it does occur, the consequences are not terrible.
- A very inappropriate thing to do – This should not be done in any circumstances, as it will make the situation worse.

When given a situational judgement question, there is a basic framework that can help you to work through it:

1. Identify the basic dilemma (in the example, it is the clash between social commitments and the need for an effective patient handover)
2. Identify your potential courses of action (where you are given options, do pick one of the options given, but also suggest an alternative action which would be better if you think there is one)
3. What qualities can be shown by each action
4. What the potential disadvantages are of these actions
5. Think about how the perspectives of colleagues/patients may differ from your own
6. Balance these to pick an action which you can justify with a sound argument

Example:
You are an FY1 on liaison psychiatry. You notice that one of the GP trainees is drinking vodka on the job with some of the patients.

Rank the actions below in the order of most appropriate to least appropriate:

A. Do nothing because they are more senior so you should not interfere
B. Notify your educational supervisor
C. Notify your clinical supervisor
D. Talk to the colleague directly
E. Contact the GMC

Stem Theme – Colleague is found drinking alcohol at work.
Examples of principles tested – Patient safety, your relationship with teammates, confidentiality of colleagues, professionalism, your duty of care to patients.
A – Good – preserves relationship with teammate; Bad – risk to patient safety, unprofessional
B – Good – action to protect patients; Bad – educational supervisor not directly involved with patient care, risk of breakdown in relationship with that GP, breach of GP's confidentiality
And so on...

> ***Top tip!*** *Always put patient safety first. If you do this, you can never go far wrong.*

MEDICAL ETHICS

There are normally multiple medical ethics questions every year so it's well worth spending your time revising them. **These principles can be applied to all cases** regardless of what social/ethnic background the healthcare professional or patient is from. The principles are:

Beneficence: The wellbeing of the patient should be the doctor's first priority. In medicine, this means that one must act in the patient's best interests to ensure the best outcome is achieved for them, i.e. 'Do Good'.

Non-Maleficence: This is the principle of avoiding harm to the patient (i.e. Do no harm). There can be a danger that in a willingness to treat, doctors can sometimes cause more harm to the patient than good. This can especially be the case with major interventions, such as chemotherapy or surgery. Where a course of action has both potential harms and potential benefits, non-maleficence must be balanced against beneficence.

Autonomy: The patient has the right to determine their own healthcare. This, therefore, requires the doctor to be a good communicator so that the patient is sufficiently informed to make their own decisions. 'Informed consent' is thus a vital precursor to any treatment. A doctor must respect a patient's refusal for treatment even if they think it is not the correct choice. Note that patients cannot demand treatment – only refuse it, e.g. an alcoholic patient can refuse rehabilitation but cannot demand a liver transplant.

There are many situations where the application of autonomy can be quite complex, for example:

- **Treating Children**: Consent is required from the parents, although the autonomy of the child is taken into account increasingly as they get older. Children younger than 18 years old can consent to treatment if they are 'Gillick Competent' but they cannot refuse it.
- **Treating adults without the capacity** to make important decisions. The first challenge with this is in assessing whether or not a patient has the capacity to make the decisions. Just because a patient has a mental illness does not necessarily mean that they lack the capacity to make decisions about their healthcare. Where patients do lack capacity, the power to make decisions is transferred to the next of kin (or Legal Power of Attorney, if one has been set up).

Justice: This principle deals with the fair distribution and allocation of healthcare resources for the population.

Consent: This is an extension of Autonomy- patients must agree to a procedure or intervention. For consent to be valid, it must be **voluntary informed consent.** This means that the patient must have sufficient mental capacity to make the decision and must be presented with all the relevant information (benefits, side effects, and the likely complications) in a way they can understand.

Confidentiality: Patients expect that the information they reveal to doctors will be kept private- this is a key component in maintaining the trust between patients and doctors. You must ensure that patient details are kept confidential. Confidentiality can be broken if you suspect that a patient is a risk to themselves or to others, e.g. Terrorism, suicides, certain infectious diseases.

MEDICAL LAW

Understanding the principles of medical law is essential when answering the questions on the SJT. Here is a brief overview of some key legal cases and principles that you should familiarise yourself with:

Mental Health Act
This act basically governs how healthcare professionals interact with people who have mental disorders and their rights to force treatment. The original act was passed in 1983, but there was a significant amendment in 2007. The most significant components for health professionals are the definition of holding powers which allow doctors to detain and treat a patient with a mental illness against their will. Most notably, these are sections 5(2) and 5(4) which define doctors' and nurses' duties respectively. Other orders to be aware of are section 135 (magistrate order) and section 136 (police order). You should hopefully have covered these during your psychiatry rotations.

Mental Capacity Act
The primary purpose of the 2005 act is to govern the decision-making process on behalf of adults who lack the capacity to make decisions for themselves. There are several principles to be aware of:

1. A person must be assumed to have the capacity unless proven otherwise.
2. A person is not to be treated as unable to make a decision unless all practicable steps to help them do so have been taken without success.
3. A person is not to be treated as unable to make a decision merely because they make an unwise decision.
4. An act must be in their best interest.
5. The act must be the least restrictive with regards to the individual's freedom.

Data Protection Act
This act gives the GMC power to control how data is collected, recorded, and used. Personal data under the act is defined as identifiable information. It's important that data is:

1) Processed fairly and lawfully
2) Gathered for specific purposes.
3) Adequate, relevant, accurate, and kept up to date

This governs how doctors collect patient information and who they can share this information with. Practical examples are doctors being allowed to break confidentiality for acts of suspected terrorism and road traffic accidents.

Gillick Competence
Children under the age of 18 can consent to treatment if they are able to understand, weigh up, and decide they want the treatment. However, they cannot refuse treatment until they are 18 years old. For children under 18 with no parent/guardian and aren't Gillick competent, you are able to act 'in their best interest'.

Bolam Test

The Bolam test is a legal rule that assesses the appropriate standard of reasonable care in negligence cases involving a skilled professional. The Bolam test states "*If a doctor reaches the standard of a responsible body of medical opinion, he is not negligent*". In order for someone to be shown as negligent, it must be established that:

1) There was a duty of care
2) The duty of care was breached

The breach directly led to the patient being harmed.

QUESTION ANSWERING STRATEGY

Treat Every Option Independently

The options may seem similar, but don't let the different options confuse you. Read each option as if it is a question of its own. It is important to know that responses should **NOT** be judged as though they are the **ONLY** thing you are to do. An answer should not be judged as inappropriate because it's incomplete, but only if there is some actual inappropriate action taking place.

For example, if a scenario says "a *patient on the ward complains she is in pain*", the response "ask the patient what is causing the problem" would be very appropriate, even though any good response would also include informing the nurses and other doctors about what you had been told.

There might be multiple correct responses for each scenario, so don't feel you have to answer each stem differently. If you are unsure of the answer, mark the question and move on. **Avoid spending more than 90 seconds on any question**, otherwise, you will fall behind and risk not finishing.

Read "Tomorrow's Doctors" and "Good Medical Practice"

These are publications produced by the General Medical Council (GMC) which can be found on their website. The GMC regulates the medical profession to ensure that standards remain high. These publications can be found on their website, and it outlines the expectations of the next generation of doctors – the generation of doctors you are aspiring to join. Reading through this will get you into a professional way of thinking and will help you to judge these questions accurately.

Step into Character

When doing this section, imagine you are in the scenarios being presented to you. Imagine yourself as the caring and conscientious junior doctor that you soon will be. What would you do? What do you think would be the right thing to do?

Hierarchy

The patient is of **primary importance**. All decisions that affect patient care should be made to benefit the patient. Of **secondary importance** are your work colleagues. So, if there is no risk to patients, you should help out your colleagues and avoid doing anything that would undermine them or harm their reputation – but if doing so would bring detriment to any patient, then the patient's priorities come to the top.

Finally, of **lowest importance** is yourself. You should avoid working outside hours and strive to further your education, but not at the expense of more important or urgent priorities. Remember the key principles of professional conduct and you cannot go far wrong. Of first and foremost importance is patient safety. Make sure you make all judgements with this hierarchy in mind.

Be Realistic

The SJT is not a knowledge-based test and the students that perform best in it tend to be ones who have substantial clinical experience. It requires you to be pragmatic when making decisions. For example, in the scenario: "An elderly gentleman from Brazil is admitted to your ward. You can't verbally communicate as you don't speak Portuguese".

In this scenario, many might consider it prudent to arrange an interpreter. However, this can be a laborious and long-winded process (especially out of standard hours). The better option, if possible, is to locate a member of staff that can speak Portuguese to interpret for you.

IMPORTANT PRINCIPLES

As mentioned previously, there are several core principles that you should attempt to apply to the questions which will aid you in ranking the answers. Most of these relate to non-technical skills, i.e. beyond knowledge based systems/theory.

Adopt a Patient-Centred Approach to Care

This involves being able to treat patients as an individual and respecting their decisions. You should also respect a patient's right to confidentiality, unless there is a significant risk to the general public (see "Good Medical Practice"). The final core tenet is maintaining patient safety. This is usually the most important one to apply during the SJT.

Working Well in a Team

Teamwork is an essential part of any job. You must be a trustworthy and reliable team member and also communicate effectively within the team, between teams, and to other specialists. You should always support your colleagues, senior or junior, should they require it. It is important to avoid conflict and be able to de-escalate situations without jeopardising professional relationships where possible.

Understanding the Limits of your Competence

This becomes more important as you progress through your training as only you will be able to assess your own competence with regards to the management of patients and in procedural skills. You should have an appreciation of what needs to be escalated, when to escalate it, and to whom.

Commitment to Professionalism

You should always act with honesty and integrity as this is expected of anyone entering the profession. This includes apologising for your mistakes and trying to ensure other people apologise for theirs.

Taking Responsibility for your learning

Medicine is a career where you are continuously learning. You are the sole person responsible for it and you will need to prioritise your jobs to ensure you attend scheduled teaching and courses. You should be able to critically reflect upon your experiences.

Top tip! *Remember, it's what you* ***SHOULD*** *do – not what you* ***WOULD*** *do.*

QUESTIONS

PRACTICE QUESTIONS

Question 1:

You are on call over the weekend and have been attending to a sick patient on one of the wards. When you arrive at the acute admissions ward the nurse in charge starts shouting angrily at you for being irresponsible. She says that you are late and should have come sooner as there are many urgent jobs to do.

Rank the actions below in order of most appropriate to least appropriate:

A. Tell the nurse that they should have bleeped you if they really needed you
B. Refuse to do any jobs until the nurse apologises
C. Tell the nurse to lodge a complaint
D. Threaten to lodge a complaint against the nurse unless they calm down
E. Explore why the nurse is so angry, explain where you have been and that you didn't realise that there were urgent jobs to do.

Question 2:

You are the FY1 on the ward round where your other FY1 colleague is running late. When she eventually turns up she says she is feeling unwell with stomach cramps and has been vomiting all morning causing her to be late. She asks you to leave the ward round to give her some IV fluids and some paracetamol from the treatment room to help her feel better so she can come help you.

Choose the **THREE** most appropriate actions to take in this situation:

A. Tell her to go home if she is feeling unwell
B. Report her to your consultant for coming in when she is an infection risk
C. Give her some of your own paracetamol
D. Tell her she needs to sort herself out quickly as the ward is very busy and you need her help
E. Give her some IV fluids to help her recover quickly as you have a lot of patients and will need her help
F. Explain that you are in the middle of the ward round and she should ask someone else for help
G. Offer to cover for the day while she recovers

Question 3:

You are the FY1 on call and have been bleeped to see a patient on a ward. Whilst there a nurse approaches you about a different patient and asks you to write up their venous thromboembolism prophylaxis after a surgery as she asked the ward FY1 to sign the prescription, but they had said they were too busy and refused to sign the prescription.

Choose the **THREE** most appropriate actions to take in this situation:

A. Speak to the doctor who refused to sign the medication
B. Complain to the nurse in charge about the nurse in question because she is undermining the decisions of the ward doctors
C. Go and see the patient in question
D. Refuse to sign the prescription and tell the nurse that there will be a good reason why the doctor she had previously ask refused
E. Speak to your consultant about your FY1 colleague as they are neglecting patient care
F. Advise the nurse to speak directly to the doctor in question in the future
G. Advise the nurse to speak to your consultant about the doctor in question

Question 4:

You are the FY1 on a surgical firm and you notice that your FY2 often takes home the patient list in order to be able to memorise the patients for the consultant ward round, which means they do not have to come in so early as you to prepare.

Rank the actions below in order of most appropriate to least appropriate:

A. Start taking your own list home so you can memorise the patients too
B. Ask the nurse in charge of the surgical ward for more confidential waste bins
C. Pointedly ask if he knows where the confidential waste bins are located
D. Inform your colleague that he should not be taking the list home
E. Explain to your consultant what he is doing

Question 5:

As the surgical FY1, your consultant has advised you that one of their private patients is coming in to your ward and has asked you to clerk them in and send their pre-operative bloods on your normal NHS shift. You already have a lot of patients to see and worry that this will take up too much of your valuable time.

Rank the actions below in order of most appropriate to least appropriate:

A. Explain to the consultant that you don't have time. However, it's fine if they reimburse you to stay later after your shift to clerk their private patient.
B. Explain the situation to one of your other consultants to ask for advice
C. Ignore your consultants message and reply later saying you were too busy with your own patients
D. Ask to speak to your consultant about the increased workload
E. Do the clerking and bloods as quickly as possible

Question 6:

You are the anaesthetic FY1 on call in your first few weeks when you are the first to arrive at a cardiac arrest where nurses are performing compressions. The medical registrar arrives and asks you to put in a chest drain as it is believed the patient has a pneumothorax, while they make the notes and timings. You have only done this once, supervised before.

Rank the actions below in order of most appropriate to least appropriate:

A. Do the chest drain yourself
B. Ask one of the nurses to bleep the FY2 to come help
C. Ask the medical registrar for guidance on performing the drain
D. Tell the registrar you can do the notes while they do the drain
E. Refuse to do the drain

Question 7:

You have been on day shifts for the past two weeks and have consistently been leaving late because your colleague working the night shift has been arriving increasingly late. You have a friend's birthday party to go to and you are about to finish your shift but your colleague has not arrived for you to handover the jobs.

Rank the actions below in order of most appropriate to least appropriate:

A. Leave a written handover in the doctors office and tell the nurses to alert your colleague to these when they arrive
B. Call personnel to see if your colleague has called in sick
C. Wait for your colleague to arrive
D. Hand over to another doctor who is just starting their night shift and ask them to relay to your colleague when they arrive
E. Call your colleague to ask where they are

Question 8:

You are the FY1 working in a sexual health clinic. You have seen the patient and they are requesting a contraceptive underarm implant. You run this by the consultant, who agrees to put in the implant. Just before starting the procedure, your consultant gets bleeped away and says that you should just do it yourself and they will be back after they have answered the bleep. You have only seen the procedure done once and have read about it in textbooks. The patient is asking you to hurry if possible as she needs to leave and does not know when she will have time to come back as she is very busy.

Choose the **THREE** most appropriate actions to take in this situation:

A. Quickly check the procedure steps online then do the implant
B. Keep the patient in the room ready in the hope that the consultant will return soon
C. Do not insert the implant but offer the patient alternative contraception to use until she can return to the clinic
D. Call you consultant and ask how long they will be
E. Explain to the patient that you can do the implant now or she can wait for the consultant to return
F. Ask one of your registrars to supervise you during the procedure
G. Do not do the procedure, the patient will have to wait
H. Perform the procedure and ask the patient to come back at the next available opportunity to have it checked

Question 9:

You are the surgical FY1 and are assisting in a Caesarean section. During the procedure your senior accidentally pricks you with a needle. There is no one else available to help assist in the operation but it is nearing the end and your consultant says they are able to finish the case alone.

Rank the actions below in order of most appropriate to least appropriate:

A. Send a sample of the patient's blood you have saved for an HIV test
B. Carry on with the operation and complete an incident form after
C. Report to occupational health immediately
D. Bleep your colleague to come and take over assisting in the operation
E. Remove your gloves and run the affected area under a tap

Question 10:

During gynaecology pre-assessment clinic you find one of your patients to have a urinary tract infection. You prescribe antibiotics and send the urine for microbiology culture. The patient tells you that it often takes a few weeks to get a GP appointment, as their practice is very busy. Several days later, the urine culture returns and shows that the infection is resistant to the antibiotic you prescribed.

Rank the actions below in order of most appropriate to least appropriate:

A. Call the patient and ask them to make an appointment with their GP
B. Send the patient's GP a letter explaining the situation
C. Tell the patient to present to their local A&E and explain the situation
D. Tell the patient to come and see you on the ward for a hospital pharmacy prescription
E. Cancel the patient's gynaecology surgery as they have a current infection

Question 11:

You are the FY1 on call at night and are called to see a patient receiving IV antibiotics and fluids for a post-surgical infection. His cannula has fallen out and you're unable to cannulate him despite two attempts in his forearm. The patient is adamant that he does not want a cannula in his hands.

Rank the actions below in order of most appropriate to least appropriate:

A. Record the unsuccessful attempts and write in their notes for their day team to review in the morning
B. Call your FY2 for help
C. Bleep the anaesthetist on call to help establish IV access
D. Change the patient's antibiotics to an oral prescription
E. Explain you have no option but to attempt a cannula in the patients' hand

Question 12:

You are the FY1 on a medical firm. The consultant asks some medical students to write a case study on a patient. You offer to let them see a case report that you've written in the past. The students submit their reports to the consultant who asks you to have a look at them. You notice that one of the students has copied your case report almost entirely and has clearly not seen the patient at all.

Choose the **THREE** most appropriate actions to take in this situation:

A. Inform the medical school what the student has done
B. Do nothing as the student may not have had time to see any patients
C. Ask your consultant what they think about copying others' work
D. Ask the student to rewrite his case report
E. Read the GMC guidelines for plagiarism
F. Ask the student about what you believe to have happened
G. Explain what has happened to the consultant
H. Explain to the students about the importance of professionalism as a doctor

Question 13:

You are working in A&E. One day in the treatment room you observe a healthcare assistant put some medications in his pocket. You worry that he may be taking them home for himself.

Rank the actions below in order of most appropriate to least appropriate:

A. Inform your consultant of what you have seen
B. Ask the healthcare assistant what he is doing with the medicines
C. Inform the personnel department that you think the healthcare assistant is stealing
D. Privately tell the healthcare assistant to put the medicines back and to go home
E. Ignore the situation as he may be taking the medicines for some patients

Question 14:

You are looking after a patient on the ward who presented with long term bloody diarrhoea and weight loss. You strongly suspect bowel cancer. One day, he calls you over and asks you directly "*Do I have Cancer Doctor?*"

Rank the actions below in order of most appropriate to least appropriate:

A. Tell your patient you are still awaiting test results but will ask your consultant to come and see him when the results are available
B. Reassure him that there is nothing to worry about you are just running a few routine tests
C. Arrange to have a discussion with your patient and leave your bleep outside
D. Explain that it is likely that he has cancer
E. Explain that you are still waiting for test results but will let him know about them as soon as possible

Question 15:

One of your colleagues comes to you one day out of work saying that she is feeling increasingly stressed and has been drinking alcohol to help her relax. She asks you not to mention this to anyone. She reassures you that she would never drink at work but is finding it increasingly difficult to cope and feels very tired at work.

Rank the actions below in order of most appropriate to least appropriate:

A. Counsel them as a friend and do not tell anyone
B. Tell your ward nurses that you think your colleague is stressed and to go easy on them with work if they can
C. Report your colleague to your hospital personnel department for inappropriate behaviour
D. Advise your colleague to speak to their clinical advisor about the stresses at work
E. Tell your consultant that you are worried about your colleague's drinking

Question 16:

You are the urology FY1 and work with an Asian registrar. A patient needs to be catheterised so your registrar goes away to collect the kit. Meanwhile, the patient tells you that he doesn't want the registrar to touch him and wants you to do the procedure instead.

Rank the actions below in order of most appropriate to least appropriate:

A. Do the catheter yourself
B. Tell your registrar the patient does not want him to do the catheter
C. Tell the patient he cannot pick his doctor
D. Explore the patient's concerns
E. Refuse to treat the patient

Question 17:

You are working in A&E when you see a young woman with bruises all over her arms who claims to have fallen over. Upon further questioning she admits that her partner is occasionally physically abusive to her but asks you to not tell anyone, as she is worried he will find out.

Choose the **THREE** most appropriate actions to take in this situation:

A. Inform her partner you know what he is doing and arrange for him to come to A&E to see you
B. Speak to your senior about what you have discovered
C. Offer the patient details of domestic abuse support groups and numbers to call in the hope she changes her mind
D. Contact the patient's GP to follow her up in a few weeks
E. Inform the police
F. Do nothing and respect her confidentiality as she is an adult with capacity
G. Call the partner and ask him to book an appointment with his GP
H. Contact the safeguarding team at your hospital for advice

Question 18:

You are one of the doctors working in A&E. A child is admitted following a serious road traffic accident and needs to be given blood urgently. The boy's parents explain that they are Jehovah's Witnesses and they do not want him to receive a blood transfusion under any circumstances as it is against their religious belief.

Choose the **THREE** most appropriate actions to take in this situation:

A. Respect the parents' wishes and try and help the boy without blood products
B. Call the hospital chaplain in an attempt to persuade the parents
C. Overrule the parent's wishes as this is an emergency situation
D. Contact one of your seniors for advice
E. Explain to the parents the seriousness of their son's condition and why he needs the transfusion
F. Tell the parents they are being irresponsible and their son will die without the transfusion
G. Ask the parents about what their son would want for himself
H. Hold the transfusion until the boy is conscious and able to consent for himself

Question 19:

You are one of the doctors at the mess party. Your registrar colleagues asks you whether your FY1 friend is single as he finds her attractive and would like to ask her on a date.

Rank the actions below in order of most appropriate to least appropriate:

A. Explain that you do not know but suggest your registrar speaks to your FY1 friend himself
B. Say that you find this behaviour inappropriate and walk away
C. Tell your registrar your FY1 friend is single and give him her phone number
D. Tell your consultant what has happened
E. Inform your FY1 friend what the registrar has said to you

Question 20:

You are the psychiatry FY1 and seeing patients in substance misuse clinic. You see a gentleman who is awaiting detox for alcohol misuse. While chatting you ascertain that he works as a lorry driver and says that he has been fine with this for many years despite his drinking. He doesn't think it impacts on his ability to drive.

Choose the **THREE** most appropriate actions to take in this situation:

A. Inform the DVLA
B. Explain to him that he must not carry on driving while drinking as it could be very dangerous
C. Do nothing as he is likely to be undertaking detox soon
D. Call his wife and explain the situation
E. Confront him and say it is irresponsible to be driving while drinking and that if he doesn't provide evidence that he has stopped driving you will call the police
F. Call the police straightaway

Question 21:

You are the FY1 in A&E. A female patient with capacity presents with vaginal bleeding. She needs an urgent speculum examination. She refuses to allow you to examine her and demands to see a more senior female doctor. You look around but none of them are available.

Rank the actions below in order of most appropriate to least appropriate:

A. Take their history and respect their request but explain that if their condition becomes critical you will need to proceed with the examination
B. Wait for a more senior female doctor to become available
C. Insist that the examination is urgent, and you will have to proceed as there are no other doctors available
D. Explain the urgent need for the examination and explain that there is no doctors matching their desired description available, but respect their request if they decline and wait for another doctor
E. Offer a female chaperone from the healthcare team as a compromise

Question 22:

You are the FY2 working on a ward. One of the patients' relatives approaches you looking distressed. They are worried about how the nurses are caring for their relative and are considering making a formal complaint. They ask for your advice.

Rank the actions below in order of most appropriate to least appropriate:

A. Tell her you will check with the team about what has been going on but a formal complaint won't make any difference
B. Explore her concerns and attempt to alleviate any misunderstandings
C. Suggest she speaks to the patient family liaison department in the hospital for advice
D. Inform your consultant and the nurses working on the ward about her concerns
E. Tell her you also have concerns about the nurses and encourage her to make a complaint

Question 23:
You are bleeped to the private ward in your hospital. When you arrive, the nurses explain that one of the patients was receiving an urgent infusion of post-operative fluids but their cannula has stopped working. When she called the consultant responsible for the patient they asked her to bleep the FY1 On call.

Rank the actions below in order of most appropriate to least appropriate:

A. Offer to help but explain that in the future they should have their own staff available to cannulate private patients
B. Contact the ward manager to ask about the staff they have available to help in these situations as you are very busy working on shift for the NHS
C. Help with the cannula but leave a note to explain that you will invoice for this work
D. Assess the patient and the situation quickly and order in your jobs list according to its priority
E. Refuse to cannulate the patient as you are already overworked with your NHS patients

Question 24:
You are in your final rotation of your FY1 year. You're working with another FY1 colleague and notice that they are unable to do ABGs which they should be able to do by now.

Rank the actions below in order of most appropriate to least appropriate:

A. Advise them to ask a senior for guidance with the issue
B. Email their clinical advisor to explain the problem
C. Offer to help them practise ABGs in the clinical skills laboratory
D. Avoid the problem until they ask you for help
E. Raise the issue in front of a patient during a ward round so they are forced to admit the problem

Question 25:
You are working as the FY1 in the sexual health clinic. Your patient has been cheating on his long-term girlfriend by having unprotected sex with another man. He is worried he has a sexually transmitted disease. On examination it is apparent that he has genital warts.

Choose the **THREE** most appropriate actions to take in this situation:

A. Tell him you must contact his girlfriend to explain her chances of having the disease
B. Advise him to have an HIV test
C. Advise him to inform his regular partner
D. Give advice about safe sexual practices
E. Test him for HIV as he is in a high risk group
F. Inform the patients' GP so they can follow up to ensure they have been adequately treated
G. Offer relationship counselling as he is clearly unhappy in his current relationship
H. Tell him you will have to contact the man he had sex with so he can get checked

Question 26:

You are the paediatrics FY1. A 10-year-old boy is admitted with abdominal pain. Whilst taking the history, the interaction between the father and son appears completely normal. However, when his father steps out of the room to take a telephone call, the boy tells you that his father sometimes hits him when he is angry.

Rank the actions below in order of most appropriate to least appropriate:

A. Do a full physical examination in the presence of the father explaining that you are looking for signs of abuse
B. Ask the father about what the boy has said, allowing him to offer an explanation for the boys' accusations
C. Make a clear documentation of what the boy say and ask him more about the incidents described
D. Call the police to report the child abuse
E. Assume that the boy is referring to reasonable discipline as he appears to be well cared for

Question 27:

You are a medical FY1. One of the patients on your ward has a DNACPR (Do not attempt cardio-pulmonary resuscitation) order in place due to terminal bowel cancer. On overhearing the patient with their relatives one day it becomes apparent that they are unaware this order is in place.

Rank the actions below in order of most appropriate to least appropriate:

A. Apologise to the patient and the family for their previous team being neglectful and not explaining the order properly
B. Explain that that the DNACPR is in place because cardiopulmonary resuscitation is unlikely to be successful to the patient and their relatives
C. Wait until you have an opportunity to discuss the order with the patient alone
D. Consider the DNACPR invalid until you have discussed it with the patient
E. Inform the seniors in the team of the situation

Question 28:

You are on a surgical attachment with another FY1 doctor. You notice that he frequently takes surgical equipment home which he claims is to practice his surgical skills.

Rank the actions below in order of most appropriate to least appropriate:

A. Tell him he should return all of the equipment as soon as possible
B. Do nothing as it will compromise patient care if your colleague doesn't practise his surgical skills
C. Inform the clinical supervisor about what you have seen
D. Tell him you will have to report him to your consultant if you see him take any more equipment
E. Inform the theatre manager about what you have seen

Question 29:

You are the FY1 on general surgery. During the ward round, the consultant and registrar are called away to attend to an emergency patient. They explain that the next patient just needs to be consented for a left hemicolectomy ready to be next on today's surgical list.

Rank the actions below in order of most appropriate to least appropriate:

A. Ask another registrar who has undertaken the operation previously to consent the patient
B. Complete all of your other urgent jobs then consent the patient
C. Explain to the registrar that you do not have enough experience to consent the patient for this operation
D. Consent the patient to the best of your ability.
E. Ask the registrar for instructions on how to consent the patient and then do so

Question 30:

You have been on a long day shift when a nurse approaches you to write the prescription for a patient you do not know. You are feeling extremely tired and hungry and finding it increasingly difficult to concentrate. You were planning to go for a break to eat something to help you feel more alert towards the end of your shift.

Choose the **THREE** most appropriate actions to take in this situation:

A. Explain to the nurse that you need a break but will attend to it as soon as you return
B. Say you are busy and to ask someone else
C. Ask her to call the on-call team to do the prescriptions
D. Write the prescription quickly then go for your break
E. Ask the nurse to fill in most of the prescription which you can then sign for her
F. Try your best to do the prescription
G. Offer to do the prescription later
H. Enquire about the urgency of the prescription

Question 31:

You have been working as an FY1 for 2 months but are still struggling with basic clinical skills such as cannulation and venepuncture. You find yourself avoiding them when possible. When you do try them, it takes such a significant amount of time that it impacts on your working day.

Choose the **THREE** most appropriate actions to take in this situation:

A. Ask your colleagues for help with doing these skills when they are required
B. Avoid patients for whom you believe it will be difficult to practise these skills
C. Realise that you are not suited to medicine and change careers
D. Take an active approach to practising in the hope that you will improve
E. Ask another more senior colleague to supervise you during a few attempts
F. Set a rule of only attempting these skills on each patient once and bleep someone more senior if you are unsuccessful
G. Change your ward patients' cannulas & take their bloods more frequently to practise
H. Ask the clinical skills director for some time in the laboratory to practise

Question 32:

You are the FY1 working on a night shift. You are bleeped to the surgical ward where the nurse in charge is very distressed. She has been assaulted by a patient who seems to be confused post-operatively and is acutely unwell. The patient is shouting and demanding to go home. They are refusing all medical help.

Choose the **THREE** most appropriate actions to take in this situation:

A. Allow the patient to leave as you cannot keep them in hospital against their will
B. Try and calm the patient down to assess them
C. Ask the psychiatry team for an assessment
D. Call the hospital security to assist with restraining the patient to prevent them from leaving
E. Ask the other nurses to help restrain the patient so you can assess them
F. Sedate the patient to allow you to fully assess them
G. Bleep the surgeon who undertook the operation
H. Move the patient to another ward

Question 33:

You are the FY1 working in the sexual health clinic. You see a 15-year-old diabetic girl who has come in because she is worried that she has a sexually transmitted infection. Investigations confirm that she has chlamydia. She does not want you to tell her parents because they are very anxious about her diabetes. She appears to be thoughtful and seems to understand the treatment involved.

Rank the actions below in order of most appropriate to least appropriate:

A. Give her the treatment without telling her parents
B. Encourage the patient to tell her parents but advise you will have to do so if she does not
C. Explore her concerns about discussing the diagnosis with her parents
D. Call her parents and explain the situation as she is underage and cannot consent
E. Refuse to give her the treatment until she returns with her parents

Question 34:

You are the FY1 on general surgery. You are asked to place a request for an abdominal CT scan after the morning ward round. You submit a request for the scan but it is rejected by the consultant radiologist who wants more clinical information. Your consultant is very busy in theatre and asked you to wait till he was finished in theatre to ask any questions.

Rank the actions below in order of most appropriate to least appropriate:

A. Ask your registrar about the information required
B. Call your consultant in theatre to ask about the information
C. Ask the radiologist to contact your consultant directly about the information
D. Make up the information that the radiologist wants which isn't available in the patient notes
E. Make a record in the patients' notes about why the scan was refused and move on to other jobs

Question 35:

You are the FY1 working on a busy surgical ward. There are significant gaps in the rota and the department is very poorly staffed. You only see your consultant for the morning ward round as they then have to go to theatre. As a consequence, you feel incredibly unsupported and have to work much longer hours than you are meant to. You frequently skip scheduled teaching. You receive no on-the-job teaching, especially compared with your other FY1 colleagues working on more supported firms.

Choose the **THREE** most appropriate actions to take in this situation:

A. Approach the consultant about the gaps in the rota and concerns about the lack of teaching
B. Attend your FY1 colleagues teaching when available and make up for the time after
C. Continue as you are- hopefully your next firm will be better
D. Complete what jobs you can but leave on time regardless
E. Complete all of your jobs but stay after work to revise from books the teaching you should be getting on the job
F. Take time off work to prevent you becoming too stressed
G. Contact your educational supervisor about the lack of learning opportunities
H. Go through your contract to ensure you are working the hours for which you are contracted and are being treated fairly

Question 36:

You are working on the care of the elderly ward for a few months. One of your patients is frequently admitted for several days due to issues with their permanent catheter. Every time they are admitted, they insist on giving you a small present such as a box of chocolates or a bottle of wine. They offer you a present on the morning ward round again.

Rank the actions below in order of most appropriate to least appropriate:

A. Ask one of your seniors to explain that they do not need to give you gifts every admission
B. Accept the gift as a token of your hard work
C. Accept the gift but explain that you will share it with the whole team on the ward
D. Sensitively refuse the gift but take it if the patient insists on you having it
E. Accept the gift and ask the patient about why they are giving it to you

Question 37:

You have been regularly working very long hours in the acute medical unit when the nurse in charge accosts you. She has just been alerted to the fact that you prescribed the incorrect dose of a medicine for a patient. Luckily, this error was noticed before the medication was given. You feel that the busy & long shifts have been making you so tired that you haven't been able to concentrate properly at work.

Rank the actions below in order of most appropriate to least appropriate:

A. Record the error in your learning portfolio and consider the reasons for its occurrence and consider how you may prevent it from happening again in the future
B. Ask to meet your supervisor for advice on the error and on the worries you have about the long shifts impacting on your work
C. Accept the responsibility for the mistake and apologise, but explain the reasons why you believe the error occurred
D. Ask the nurse to not report the error and promise you will not make a mistake again
E. Tell the nurse that the long hours are causing you to make mistakes

Question 38:

You are the endocrinology FY1 and are bleeped to see a patient with hypomagnesaemia. You recall very little about this condition and are unsure how to manage this patient.

Rank the actions below in order of most appropriate to least appropriate:

A. Use the internet to research the condition on a search engine
B. Assess the patient then discuss with the medical registrar as to how to proceed
C. Prescribe magnesium
D. Check your trust guidelines for any guidance on the condition
E. Bleep the medical registrar for advice

Question 39:

You are coming to the end of your surgical FY1 rotation. You have found it to be incredibly stressful and unsupported. You feel that your induction didn't prepare you for the difficulties involved. You want to help the incoming doctors prepare for this difficult rotation.

Rank the actions below in order of most appropriate to least appropriate:

A. Explain to your clinical supervisor about the difficulties you faced and any advice on how to improve the rotation
B. Take time off during your next rotation to help your successor
C. Make a list of advice for your successor
D. Ensure the next doctor has your phone number so they can contact you for advice
E. Hope that the induction process will be improved for your successor

Question 40:

You have a patient on the ward with long standing Parkinson's disease. You notice that they haven't received their normal medications for the past three days. The patient's nurse states that the patient has been refusing their medication. In your experience, the patient always appears to be very cooperative and willing to take on medical advice. When you ask the patient about the medications they deny being offered medications by the nurse.

Rank the actions below in order of most appropriate to least appropriate:

A. Change all of the patient medicines into the intravenous forms
B. Check the patients' memory ability regarding other activities on the ward
C. Report the nurse to the Royal College of Nursing
D. File an incident report against the nurse for failing to give the medications
E. Explain the situation to the ward sister and ask her to investigate

Question 41:

During your cardiology rotation, you become worried as notice that your registrar often misses basic signs such as arrhythmias and murmurs. You politely suggest this to your consultant one day but he dismisses it by saying that the registrar "is an excellent teacher and you could learn a lot from him".

Rank the actions below in order of most appropriate to least appropriate:

A. Ask you consultant again to consider the registrars' clinical skills and ability to detect signs
B. Ask your educational supervisor for advice
C. Inform the head of the cardiology department
D. Approach your registrar and tell him your concerns and offer to teach him about the signs he has been missing
E. Review all the patients yourself after the registrar has completed their ward round.

Question 42:

You are working on a gastroenterology ward. One of the nurses approaches you and says that she gave the wrong dose of a drug this morning to a patient and has only just realised her mistake. She is worried about the patient and asks you to not let anyone else know about her mistake.

Choose the **THREE** most appropriate actions to take in this situation:

A. Go and assess the patient if they appear well avoid documenting in the notes about the incident
B. Call your consultant to have the nurse removed from the ward
C. Go and assess the patient in question urgently
D. Go and asses the patient and tell them to not take their next dose of the drug
E. Tell the nurse to fix the situation herself otherwise you will have to report it
F. Explain that you have to inform the nurse in charge about the mistake
G. Make a formal report about the incident
H. Write in the notes about the mistake

Question 43:

You are working on your paediatrics rotation. You see a baby who you suspect is being physically abused. When you question the mother sensitively, she breaks down into tears and admits that her husband is physically abusing her and the baby. She does not want to seek help as she has no financial means of supporting herself and the child without him.

Choose the **THREE** most appropriate actions to take in this situation:

A. Contact social services, even if it is without the mothers' consent as the child is at risk
B. Respect the mothers' wishes and make a note in the child's file
C. Contact the partner and advise him to seek professional help
D. Call the police
E. Inform one of your senior colleagues
F. Give the mother contact details for local domestic abuse services and advise her to contact them if she changes her mind
G. Deliberately delay the child's treatment so that mother and child can stay at the hospital for longer
H. Admit the child to give you time to persuade the mother to seek help

Question 44:

You are one of two FY1 doctors on a busy medical ward. Two weeks into the rotation, you notice that your FY1 colleague consistently only takes on a small number of jobs and works very slowly.

Choose the **THREE** most appropriate actions to take in this situation:

A. Ask your colleague to stay later to make up the time wasted during the day
B. Arrange to discuss the situation with your colleague as this cannot continue
C. Speak to your other FY1s explain how unfair the situation is
D. Work harder to compensate as they may just getting used to the job
E. Wait for your seniors to notice the disparity in your work
F. Discuss with the nurses on the ward and ask them to give your colleague more of the work
G. Discuss with your seniors what has been going on

Question 45:

You are at the doctors' mess party when you accidentally overhear two FY1s talking about a night out last week. One of them received a police caution for a fairly innocuous drunken offence but they reveal that they won't inform anyone about it.

Rank the actions below in order of most appropriate to least appropriate:

A. Pretend you did not overhear the conversation as the offence will not impact patient care
B. Talk to the FY1 in question after the party about the GMC guidance regarding cautions
C. Apologise to the FY1 but explain that you will have to tell the GMC
D. Speak to the other FY1 to ascertain more information about the event
E. Organise a meeting with the FY1 welfare supervisor to discuss what you overheard

Question 46:

You are the gynaecology FY1 and assisting your registrar during an exploratory laparoscopy. During the procedure, you observe the registrar accidently clip one of the uterine arteries. You raise this with the registrar who explains that he will remove the clip later. However, you are now close to the end of the operation and are confident that the clip is still in place.

Rank the actions below in order of most appropriate to least appropriate:

A. Leave the theatre and contact your consultant asking him to come to the theatre immediately
B. Realise you must have missed the removal of the clip and revise the steps of the operation later
C. Allow the registrar to close then raise the issue with them after the operation
D. Insist to the registrar that you are confident the clip is still in place and it is a mistake
E. Ask the consultant anaesthetist to help with the situation

Question 47:

You are the FY2 on a morning ward. The consultant explains that he cannot continue as he has a headache. He asks the nurse to get him some codeine from the ward medicine room.

Rank the actions below in order of most appropriate to least appropriate:

A. Do nothing as you will not be able to do the ward round by yourself
B. Explain to the nurse that she should not allow doctors to take medicines from the ward
C. Make a report about the incident after the ward round
D. Offer to make the consultant an outpatient prescription for the codeine
E. Tell the consultant that they should go to the urgent care centre to have the codeine formally prescribed

Question 48:

You are one of the doctors working on the labour ward. A pregnant lady is admitted and urgently needs a Caesarean section as the monitors show that the baby is very distressed. She refuses to consent to a Caesarean section unless her own life is at risk and asks for analgesia because she is in significant pain.

Rank the actions below in order of most appropriate to least appropriate:

A. Respect her wishes and try and help without the operation
B. Tell her that she is likely to die without the operation
C. Explain the risks of not having the operation to her
D. Ask her partner to persuade her to have the operation
E. Perform the operation without her consent as she has lost capacity

Question 49:

You are the FY1 on a ward. A patient is very distressed because her wedding ring has gone missing. Later, when you are finishing your shift, one of your colleagues drops their bag and a ring similar to the one your patient describes falls out.

Rank the actions below in order of most appropriate to least appropriate:

A. Ask your colleague about the situation to see if she did steal the ring
B. Call the police
C. Tell your patient to ask your colleague if she knows where the ring is
D. As your colleague if she took the ring from your patient
E. Tell your consultant what has happened

Question 50:

You are working in A&E. You see a patient who is under police arrest for disorderly behaviour. When the patient is ready for discharge, the police officers ask for a copy of the medical report. The patient refuses to give permission for the police officers to have the report but the officers demand a copy.

Rank the actions below in order of most appropriate to least appropriate:

A. Discuss the situation with your seniors
B. Tell the police officers that you are completely forbidden from breaking a patient's confidentiality
C. Give a copy of the report to the patient so the officers can take it directly from him if they wish
D. Explain to the officers than you cannot give them a copy without the patients' consent
E. Give the officers a copy of the report

Question 51:

You are the FY1 in obstetrics and gynaecology. You're assisting in an emergency Caesarean section. The patient is under general anaesthetic. You successfully deliver the baby but upon inspection notice that there is an aggressive tumour in the uterus. The safest thing is to remove the whole uterus immediately, but this would obvious impact the patient's future fertility. The woman's' husband is outside with the baby.

Rank the actions below in order of most appropriate to least appropriate:

A. Explain the situation to the husband and ask him what he thinks his wife would want
B. Explain the situation to the husband and ask for his consent to perform the hysterectomy
C. Explain to the senior conducting the operation you would be unhappy to proceed with any further intervention as the patient has not consented
D. Advise the senior performing the operation to send a sample of the suspicious lesion to check the histology
E. Assist the senior with the hysterectomy as it is in the best interests of the patient

Question 52:

You are the endocrinology FY1 have just finished your day shift. You're on your way home to a friends' birthday party. En route, you remember that you have forgotten to prescribe a hormone for one of your patients for tomorrow morning. The hormone is time sensitive but was only added to their medicines today. You have called the overnight on-call FY1 on their mobile but haven't managed to get through.

Choose the **THREE** most appropriate actions to take in this situation:

A. Come in early tomorrow morning to prescribe the hormone
B. Call the ward and tell them to bleep the overnight on-call FY1 with the information and to call you back if there are any problems
C. Head back to the hospital to prescribe the hormone
D. Go to your friends' birthday party but after go back to the hospital
E. Call the FY1 every hour until you manage to speak to them to prescribe the hormone
F. Send a text to the on-call FY1 with the patients' information and the prescription required
G. Call one of the nurses on the ward and ask them to give the hormone in the morning you can write up the prescription when you start your shift
H. Call the on-call medical registrar to prescribe the hormone

Question 53:

You are the paediatrics FY1. Your registrar is running behind on an audit deadline and asks you to hold his bleep for the day so he can work on the audit. He will remain in the hospital throughout the day.

Choose the **THREE** most appropriate actions to take in this situation:

A. Refuse to take the bleep as you do not have enough experience to hold it for them
B. Accept the bleep but contact the registrar when you need help
C. Call your consultant to ask for advice
D. Refuse to take the bleep but ask the nurses to contact you wherever possible to reduce the workload for your registrar
E. Ask your registrar to give the bleep to another registrar of the same grade
F. Accept the bleep and check with your consultant when you need help
G. Accept the bleep but explain that you can only do this for a day to help out
H. Accept the bleep and consult with your other FY1 colleagues for advice

Question 54:
You are working in the sexual health clinic. Your next patient is a 14 year old girl and wants the contraceptive pill as she is in a relationship.

Choose the **THREE** most appropriate actions to take in this situation:

A. Refuse to prescribe her the pill
B. Report the patient to the police as she is engaging in sexual activity underage
C. Ask about the patients' relationship to ensure she is not being abused
D. Tell her you will have to inform her parents
E. Encourage her to tell her parents about her relationship
F. Inform social services
G. Tell the patient she will need to return with her parents to consent for her
H. Explain the need for additional measures to protect against sexually transmitted diseases and prescribe the pill

Question 55:
You are coming to the end of your FY2 rotation in psychiatry. One of the patients who you have regularly treated for alcohol addiction to is being discharged. She gives you a thank you card and her contact details. She asks you to get in touch so you can be friends outside of work.

Rank the actions below in order of most appropriate to least appropriate:

A. Explain that because of the nature of their admission it would be inappropriate to have any sort of relationship
B. Explain that they are welcome to send details of how they are getting on to your hospital, but that you cannot use your personal contact information
C. Give the patient your contact details so they can get in touch
D. Inform the consultant psychiatrist of the situation
E. Tell the patient you will contact them after they have are fully recovered and are no longer under the care of a psychiatry team

Question 56:
You are working on a geriatrics ward where one of your patients is being discharged. As they are leaving, they try to give you an expensive bottle of Champagne to say thank you. You have only met them a few times.

Choose the **THREE** most appropriate actions to take in this situation:

A. Explain that such a gift is not necessary
B. Refuse, as such a gift is out of proportion to the care provided
C. Accept the gift and say thank you so as to not cause offence
D. Accept the Champagne but explain you will share it with the other doctors
E. Ask the patient about why they are giving you the gift
F. Accept the Champagne but explain you will share it with the nursing staff
G. Accept the Champagne but explain they do not need to give gifts for their care
H. Ask your consultant to accept the Champagne on your behalf

Question 57:

You are working as the FY1 on an endocrinology firm. You see a patient with moderate learning difficulties and long-term endocrine syndrome-related problems that require them to take many medications at specific times. They are distressed as they struggle to remember to take the medicines are the right time and ask if they can take fewer medications.

Choose the **THREE** most appropriate actions to take in this situation:

A. Tell the patient to book an appointment with their GP
B. Go through their medicines and explain why they need to take each one and make them a clear medicine timetable
C. Tell the patient to try their hardest to take them at the right times but it is okay if they don't always stick to the exact timings
D. Contact their GP to explain the situation and ask them to explain the medicines to the patient
E. Review the patient's drug chart to see if there are any medications that can be stopped. Speak with your consultant before stopping them
F. Explain the situation to your registrar and explore the possibility of getting specialist external help like learning disability specialty nurses
G. Arrange a carer for the patient as they are unable to cope at home
H. Stop all non-critical medications like steroids and synthetic hormones as they are unlikely to offer benefit in this case
I. Ask the patient to speak to the nurse who conducts the daily ward drug rounds

Question 58:

You are working in A&E and looking after a patient with chest pain. After a long discussion, your consultant asks you to order a head CT scan to which you agree to. However, after reviewing the patient, you firmly believe the CT is not necessary and would be exposing the patient to unnecessary radiation.

Rank the actions below in order of most appropriate to least appropriate:

A. Refuse to book the CT scan
B. Go back to the consultant and ask what the scan is for
C. Tell the consultant that you do not agree with the scan
D. Order the scan but tell the radiologist that you do not agree with it
E. Ask an A&E registrar about the case and if they know why the consultant has ordered the scan

Question 59:

You are working on a respiratory ward. A healthcare assistant approaches you nervously as they accidentally sustained a needle stick injury yesterday. She was too embarrassed to say anything at the time but has since realised that it could be very dangerous and would like your help.

Rank the actions below in order of most appropriate to least appropriate:

A. Tell her to contact the patient from whom the blood was being taken yesterday
B. Tell her to wash the injury area immediately and milk the site
C. Tell her to go to occupational health for advice
D. Advise her to avoid any procedures where she may be exposed to other patient's blood for the time being
E. Report her to the ward sister

Question 60:

You are working on a care of the elderly ward. A patient is admitted with reduced mobility. She seems and is adamant that she does not want to be in hospital. She desperately wants to go home. Her family are asking you to ignore her wishes and give her all the treatment necessary.

Rank the actions below in order of most appropriate to least appropriate:

A. Perform a memory assessment
B. Do not discharge her as the family are acting in the patients' best interests
C. Give supportive treatment to the patient but let her go home
D. Respect the patients' wishes and let her go home
E. Ask your consultant for advice

Question 61:

You are covering a locum shift as an FY1 in your normal hospital but on an unfamiliar ward. A patients' family member demands to know what is happening with their relatives' care. It's unclear from the notes what the management plan is and none of their normal team are working today.

Choose the **THREE** most appropriate actions to take in this situation:

A. Ask your normal consultant for advice
B. Tell the relative to ask their normal team
C. Telephone a member of the team who normally looks after the patient
D. Ask the patient for consent to share their medical information with their relative
E. Explain to the family member that you are covering and aren't quite sure of the management plan but will let them know when you have found out more information
F. Ask the nurses for information on the patient and explain what you can to the relative
G. Tell the relative as much information as you have
H. Refuse to give the relative any information

Question 62:

You are in your FY2 rotation in general practice. One of the patients who you have regularly seen gives you their business card with their contact details. They ask you to keep in contact as they have enjoyed getting to know you.

Rank the actions below in order of most appropriate to least appropriate:

A. Tell the patient you will contact them if they change to another doctor
B. Tell the patient that any relationship outside the professional environment would mean you can no longer treat them
C. Agree to let them know how you are getting on, so as to not cause offence but then don't contact them
D. Agree to contact the patient
E. Ask one of the GPs for advice

Question 63:

You are the surgical FY1. On the morning ward round, your consultant informs you that a certain post-operative patient can go home. When you return later, you are worried as they look unwell. The patient is keen to go home and there is already bed assigned to another incoming patient.

Rank the actions below in order of most appropriate to least appropriate:

A. Ask your consultant to come and reassess the patient
B. Ask a consultant from another team to assess the patient
C. Ask your registrar to come assess the patient
D. Keep the patient in hospital for another day to be sure
E. Let the patient go home

Question 64:

You have just started your second medical FY1 rotation. After a few weeks you notice that the SHO on your team often gives the wrong treatment advice to patients to the extent that you now frequently have to check their advice against the hospital guidelines. This has become increasingly time-consuming.

Rank the actions below in order of most appropriate to least appropriate:

A. Share your concerns with your educational supervisor
B. Continue to check the hospital guidelines against the SHO's advice
C. Share your concerns with the SHO in question
D. Share your concerns with the nursing staff on your ward to see if they have any more information
E. Share your concerns with your consultant

Question 65:

You are working as an FY2 on your general practice rotation. One of your patients is very worried they suffer from high blood pressure. They would like you to prescribe them some beta-blockers. You check their blood pressure and find that it is within the normal range, but they still insist on getting the beta-blockers.

Rank the actions below in order of most appropriate to least appropriate:

A. Explain that they do not need beta-blockers but offer for them to see another doctor if they are still insistent
B. Prescribe him the drug as it is unlikely to cause harm and they are clearly anxious
C. Refuse to prescribe the medication as they do not need it
D. Give them a few beta blocker tablets and book an appointment to follow up in a week
E. Explore the reasons why they want the medication and explain that they do not need it at present

Question 66:

You are working on a care of the elderly ward. A patient is admitted with increasing confusion. She is shouting that she wants to go home but her family insist she is not herself and has been acting very erratically.

Rank the actions below in order of most appropriate to least appropriate:

A. Perform a Mini-Mental State Examination (MMSE)
B. Ask the seniors on your team consultant for advice
C. Discharge the patient as she is refusing treatment
D. The family are acting in the patients' best interests and so can consent for the patients' treatment
E. Ask the family for more information and send the patient for a head CT

Question 67:

You have left work for the evening and are at a friends' birthday when you realise that you forgot to check over the bloods of a patient you ordered late in the day.

Rank the actions below in order of most appropriate to least appropriate:

A. Call the on-call team to ask them to check the blood result
B. Go back to hospital to check on the result
C. Decide that if there was any serious problem with the blood results someone would have called you
D. Develop a system for the future to ensure you do not forget such jobs again
E. Make a reminder for yourself so that you check the bloods in the morning

Question 68:

You are the on-call FY1 and have been on a long day shift. When you are handing over your remaining jobs to the night on-call FY1, they flat-out refuse to accept some of them as they state that they should have been completed in the day shift.

Rank the actions below in order of most appropriate to least appropriate:

A. Make a clear note that the FY1 refused to accept the jobs and go home
B. Report the FY1 to the GMC for compromising patient care
C. Contact your educational supervisor the next day to explain the situation
D. Apologise but explain you did not have time to do the jobs during the day
E. Stay to complete the urgent jobs that cannot wait until tomorrow.

Question 69:

You are the on-call surgical FY1. You are bleeped to see one of the patients on your list because their chest drain has fallen out and you are asked to put it back in. You have never done this before but there are no other doctors around.

Rank the actions below in order of most appropriate to least appropriate:

A. Explain calmly to the nurse in charge that you are not familiar with the procedure and that you need help
B. Refuse to help as you do not know how to do the procedure
C. Find a doctor from another ward who is familiar with the procedure and ask them to supervise you
D. Read about the procedure and then attempt it
E. Try your best with the procedure but document clearly that you were not completely sure what to do and that you were acting in the patient's best interests

Question 70:

You realise that since you have started working, you have been drinking more alcohol than normal. You don't think it is a problem until you attend the next doctors mess party where a few of your colleagues make jokes that you are a big drinker.

Choose the **THREE** most appropriate actions to take in this situation:

A. Think carefully about when you drink and consider cutting down
B. Tell your colleagues it is inappropriate for them to comment on your drinking habits
C. Use a CAGE screen to determine if you should be worried about your drinking
D. See your GP about your drinking
E. Ask one of your friends if they think you drink too much
F. Book an appointment with your educational supervisor to discuss your drinking habits
G. Stop drinking to see if you develop signs of withdrawal
H. Ask your colleagues to apologise for undermining your professional integrity

Question 71:

A senior nurse on the ward asks you to sign a prescription for some fluids that she gave earlier. You ask about why the fluids were given but she gets annoyed and says that she was doing the best for the patient. She states that there were no doctors around to sign the prescription and that no one has questioned her decisions before.

Rank the actions below in order of most appropriate to least appropriate:

A. Sign the prescription
B. Check that the correct amount of fluid was given and there were no contraindications
C. Tell the nurse that only doctors are allowed to prescribe fluids
D. Explain to the nurse that she should ask someone who is allowed to prescribe before given any sort of medicines before giving them in the future
E. Assess the patient and make a note of the fluids being given in the notes

Question 72:

You are working in general practice. You see a patient who is having a general check-up for you to sign a document for their private health insurance. He is significantly overweight but asks you to not mention this on the form as he is planning on losing weight. He will lodge a complaint against you if you refuse.

Rank the actions below in order of most appropriate to least appropriate:

A. Refuse to do the document as the patient is threatening you
B. Refuse to fill in the document if you are being asked to remove unfavourable information
C. Send the report with all of the details as the patient has asked for it to be done and so had provided consent
D. Advise the patient to ask another doctor to get a second opinion
E. Explain to the patient that you will give him a copy of the document to have when you send it

Question 73:

You cover a day shift for another FY1 who calls in sick. That evening you go to a pub for a friend's birthday where you see the FY1 who called in sick that day.
Rank the actions below in order of most appropriate to least appropriate:

A. Say nothing this time as your colleague is normally very hard working and is unlikely to do it again
B. Report the doctor to the GMC.
C. Tell you colleague you won't say anything as long as he buys you a drink
D. Discuss what you have seen with your consultant the next day
E. Go up to the FY1 and ask about why he called in sick, and tell him you will report him if he does it again

Question 74:

You are working on a ward that is particularly short staffed with nurses so you are helping out with other duties such as giving out medication. You go to take a medicine from the cabinet when you realise that the entire box is out of date. You think you used a medicine from the box for a patient yesterday without checking the expiry date.

Rank the actions below in order of most appropriate to least appropriate:

A. Tell the patient about the mistake and complete an incident form
B. Tell the patient that they received the expired medication by accident
C. Tell the ward manager what has occurred immediately
D. Check the patient from yesterday's drug chart to check the medicine against the current box
E. Do not tell the patient but document in their notes that they received expired medicine

Question 75:

You are working in the infectious diseases ward. You see a patient who has been cheating on his wife with another man. The patient is HIV positive and has not told his wife about this and has no plans to do so.

Rank the actions below in order of most appropriate to least appropriate:

A. Ask for senior help
B. Tell the patient that you will have to tell his wife if he does not
C. Tell the patient that you are going to break his confidentiality
D. Do nothing as you cannot break confidentiality
E. Try and persuade the patient to tell his wife about his HIV status

Question 76:

You are the FY1 on-call on a particularly busy shift. You are finding yourself increasingly overloaded with tasks when a patients' family approach you and ask to discuss their case in detail. You attempt to do this but find yourself becoming increasingly frustrated and angry.

Choose the **THREE** most appropriate actions to take in this situation:

A. Ask the nurses to talk to family members for the rest of the shift
B. Decide not to speak to any more family members during this shift as it will add to your stress
C. Document the discussion then go home as you are very stressed and cannot continue to work
D. Take a short break after speaking with the relatives to calm down
E. Reassess your tasks and prioritise them as well as consider what factors led to you becoming angry
F. Ask one of your colleagues to help you with your tasks
G. Apologise to the family and explain that you are very busy with other patients so they don't complain
H. Ask one of the final year medical students to take on your more time-consuming tasks

Question 77:

You are re-writing a patients' drug chart. You notice that your consultant prescribed a medication to be given three times a day although it is normally only given once every day. The patient has received a few days of medicine already and you are unsure whether the extra medicine is for a good reason.

Rank the actions below in order of most appropriate to least appropriate:

A. Tell the patient that they have been receiving the wrong dose of the medicine
B. Ask the nurses on your ward whether the consultant has written up any wrong prescriptions recently
C. Leave the dose as it is currently but attempt to contact the consultant to check the error
D. Change the prescription to one daily
E. Contact the consultant directly to check if the change in the medicine was on purpose

Question 78:

You are working as the gynaecology FY1 in theatres. A nurse calls you to see one of the patients on the list that doesn't want her hysterectomy for troublesome fibroids. The team is all in theatre getting ready to operate on the patient.

Rank the actions below in order of most appropriate to least appropriate:

A. Remind the patient that they have previously consented for the surgery and it is too late to cancel it now
B. Tell the patient you will respect their wishes and cancel the surgery
C. Attempt to move the patient further down the list to try and persuade them to have the surgery
D. Explore the reasons why the patient is refusing the surgery
E. Inform your seniors that the patient no longer wants the surgery

Question 79:

You are working on a care of the elderly ward. One of your patients passes away and the consultant asks you to put the cause of death as gastroenteritis on the death certificate. You were closely involved in their care and do not agree that this was the primary cause. The bereavement office has just called you and they want to come down immediately to complete the death certificate.

Rank the actions below in order of most appropriate to least appropriate:

A. Call the coroners' office for advice
B. Refuse to complete the death certificate
C. Go down to complete the death certificate but fill in with what you believe to be the correct information
D. Discuss the case with your registrar on the ward
E. Write the cause as your consultant advised

Question 80:
You are the on-call FY1 and are bleeped to a patient because the nurse looking after him is concerned about his fluid status. When you see the unconscious elderly patient, he looks very dry and you want to prescribe some fluids. However, the patients' family say that the patient is under the palliative care team and they do not want any more medicines as they do not want him to suffer anymore.

Rank the actions below in order of most appropriate to least appropriate:

A. Insist that the fluids do not contravene their palliative status as your do not want to be accused of allowing a patient to suffer
B. Check all of the patient notes and record to become more aware of the patients' conditions and the treatment that should be offered
C. Contact a senior doctor for advice
D. Stop all of the patient's medicines to respect the family's decision
E. Explain that without the fluids the patient is likely to suffer, and ask the family to reconsider but agree to not give them if they still don't agree

Question 81:
You are working as an FY2 in paediatrics. You see a child who has some cuts and bruises that her mother says are from play-fighting with her sibling, but you suspect non-accidental injury.

Rank the actions below in order of most appropriate to least appropriate:

A. Ask for more details from the mother about how the injuries were sustained
B. Ask the mother whether she inflicted the injuries
C. Document what you can and ask the family's GP to follow up in two weeks
D. Contact social services
E. Contact your seniors for advice

Question 82:
You are seeing a patient in Rheumatology clinic with rheumatoid arthritis. He has read about new medications and asks to be put on these to control his arthritis. The guidelines state that they need to have tried methotrexate for a defined period of time before they can be started on these, which they have not yet completed.

Rank the actions below in order of most appropriate to least appropriate:

A. Explore the patients ideas about the new medicine and explain the guidelines
B. Tell the patient they must complete a defined period of time before they can be started on the drug
C. Explain that he needs to carry on his treatment plan
D. Explain that the new treatments are unlikely to help him at this point
E. Explain that the new drug is too expensive to give to him

Question 83:
You are working in A&E and see a patient who reports to have severe chest pain. You assess the patient and send off the necessary bloods to check for a myocardial infarction or other chest pathology. You have prescribed paracetamol but are not entirely convinced that the patient is experiencing quite such a severe pain as they describe and their story does not seem to fit. You also note that this is their 24th attendance this year. They are asking for more pain relief.

Rank the actions below in order of most appropriate to least appropriate:

A. Ask for senior advice
B. Refuse to prescribe any more pain relief
C. Report the patient to the police for drug seeking behaviour
D. Record the request in the notes and make a note to review the patients' pain in an hour
E. Prescribe more paracetamol

Question 84:
You are the FY1 in geriatrics. A patient is scheduled for a hysteroscopy to investigate their post-menopausal bleeding tomorrow but they no longer want to go through with the procedure.

Rank the actions below in order of most appropriate to least appropriate:

A. Ask a member of the patient's family to consent to the procedure as it is in the patient's best interests
B. Explain the potential risks of not doing the procedure
C. Check the patient's capacity for this decision by doing an assessment
D. Respect the patient's wishes and cancel the procedure
E. Perform the procedure in the patient's best interests

Question 85:
You are coming to the end of a long on-call night shift. You are handing over to your day colleague and have five minutes until your shift finishes when you receive a bleep.

Rank the actions below in order of most appropriate to least appropriate:

A. Ignore the bleep until you have handed over all other information then answer it
B. Answer the bleep and assess the situation
C. Answer the bleep and complete whatever the task requested is
D. Answer the bleep but ask them to call back in 15 minutes when the new doctor on-call will be ready
E. Ignore the bleep but make a note of it in your handover

Question 86:

You are seeing a patient in headache clinic who frequently presents with migraines demanding investigations. This time they say the pain is under control but ask for a head CT scan. You do not think this is indicated as they have already had one previously which revealed no abnormalities and they have not mentioned any different or sinister symptoms.

Rank the actions below in order of most appropriate to least appropriate:

A. Take a more detailed history asking for more information about the headaches and specifically asking about symptoms suggesting sinister causes
B. Explore the patient's ideas and concerns about their migraines
C. Write a prescription for strong analgesia
D. Explain that the scans' risks outweigh the potential benefits
E. Clearly document about the request and the reasons you have refused it

Question 87:

You are working on a haematology firm and are looking after a patient who has been having a painful crisis. She tells you she wishes to lodge a complaint against one of the nurses. She claims she was not given her pain relief medication until you were on the ward.

Choose the **THREE** most appropriate actions to take in this situation:

A. Tell the patient that you will deal with the nurse
B. Ask the patient not to make the complaint
C. Escalate to the ward manager explaining the situation
D. Explain the complaints procedure to the patient
E. Ask one of your seniors for advice
F. Chastise the nurse for putting her patients through pain unnecessarily
G. Tell the nurse to apologise to the patient
H. Tell the ward sister about the patient's concerns but do not take the matter any further

Question 88:

You are working as the FY1 in a busy A&E department. Some of the final year medical students approach you asking for advice. They say that there is nothing useful going on in the department. Since they don't receive any teaching they would rather go home and do book-work for their approaching final exams.

Rank the actions below in order of most appropriate to least appropriate:

A. Offer to teach them
B. Offer to give them time off to do book work
C. Ask them to shadow one of the other doctors as they may have more time to teach them
D. Relay their concerns to one of the consultants so they can try to rectify the situation
E. Tell them you understand but the department is the best place to prepare for the exams

Question 89:

You are working in a general practice. You are seeing a child with an ear infection. Further questioning of the mother reveals that the child has not had any of their routine immunisations.

Rank the actions below in order of most appropriate to least appropriate:

A. Explore the reasons for why the patient has not had their vaccinations
B. Explain the benefits of vaccinations to the mother and attempt to allay any concerns she may have
C. Attend to the patient's ear infection
D. Tell the mother that the lack of vaccinations has probably led to the child's current problem
E. Refuse to treat the child until they have had their vaccinations

Question 90:

You are reviewing one of your patients after the weekend. You note that the on-call doctors prescribed a medication for one of your patients to which they are allergic. They have already had the drug for two days.

Rank the actions below in order of most appropriate to least appropriate:

A. Inform the sister on the ward about the mistake
B. Complete an incident form
C. Stop the medication
D. Assess the patient
E. Find the nurse who administered the drug and chastise them for not checking the patients allergies against the medication

Question 91:

You are working in oncology clinic. You see an elderly gentleman who speaks very limited English; his son offers to translate. Unfortunately, the prognosis is not very good for the patient, but you begin to suspect the son is not relaying all the information you are trying to give.

Rank the actions below in order of most appropriate to least appropriate:

A. Explain to the son that you need him to translate exactly what you say
B. Ask one of the healthcare assistants who speaks a similar language to translate
C. Arrange for another appointment with an interpreter present
D. Try to ascertain from the patient whether they are happy for their son to translate the consultation
E. Ask the son to leave and attempt to communicate the consultation without an interpreter

Question 92:

You are working as the surgical FY1. A nurse approaches you and says that you are dressed inappropriately and are wearing too much jewellery.

Choose the **THREE** most appropriate actions to take in this situation:

A. Tell your consultant that the nurse was being unprofessional
B. Ask your other colleagues about whether you are dressing appropriately for work
C. Remove any jewellery that conflicts with your hospital's guidelines
D. Explain that your consultant also wears as much jewellery as she likes
E. Explain that you are a good doctor and that your clinical acumen is more important than what you wear
F. Refuse to see any of the nurse's patients as they have insulted you
G. Explain that it is more difficult for you to fit with the guidelines as you do not wear uniforms like the nurses do
H. Explain that you did not realise that you were dressed inappropriately and that you will take this into account for tomorrow

Question 93:

You are working in general practice. You see an 18-month-old baby who has a viral cold with their mother. The mother is very worried about the baby and asks you prescribe a course of antibiotics.

Rank the actions below in order of most appropriate to least appropriate:

A. Explain that antibiotics are not helpful but offer advice on how to help with the baby's symptoms
B. Explore the reasons for the mother's concern and reiterate that antibiotics will not help with a virus
C. Ask the mother if there are problems at home
D. Do not prescribe the antibiotics as it may make the baby worse
E. Refuse to prescribe the antibiotics but advise the mother to return if the baby does not improve after a week or becomes worse

Question 94:

You are working on a care of the elderly ward. You are asked to take routine bloods on a patient due to be discharged, and these show that the patient has a mild hyponatraemia. You reassess the patient and they seem well and are keen to go home.

Rank the actions below in order of most appropriate to least appropriate:

A. Discharge the patient but detail the blood result in the letter to their GP
B. Explain what the bloods show to the patient and explain what options are available
C. As your consultant has requested, discharge the patient
D. Keep the patient in for another day
E. Discuss the result with your registrar

Question 95:

You are working on a general medical ward. One of your patients has had repeated emergency admissions because they don't follow the information about their blood pressure tablets. They have just been readmitted with similar problems.

Rank the actions below in order of most appropriate to least appropriate:

A. Provide her with leaflets about her medical problems so she can read the information
B. Ask the patients family to intervene to help her take her medications
C. Treat her current problem and discharge without any further advice as you have tried to explain the problems before without any success
D. Treat the patient for her current problems and arrange for follow up
E. Explain to the patient the impact of her choices on her health

Question 96:

You have been helping one of your consultants with an audit that you hope to develop into a publication. They have asked to see the results tomorrow afternoon. You have stayed up late to finish the data analysis but it almost the morning. You still haven't finished and you need to go in for an early for the morning ward round.

Choose the **THREE** most appropriate actions to take in this situation:

A. Ask one of your colleagues to help you with the data analysis
B. Stay up to finish the presentation and call in sick for the morning
C. Tell your consultant that you have not finished the data analysis as you have been very busy
D. Stay up to finish as much as you can
E. Ask your consultant to finish the remaining parts of the audit
F. Tell the consultant you have had personal problems which have prevented you from finishing analysing the data
G. Give your consultant an update on what you have done so far and explain how much longer you need to complete the work
H. Go to bed now and finish the work when you have free time tomorrow

Question 97:

Your consultant turns up to the morning ward round for the third day in a row looking untidy and smelling of alcohol. You are the only member of the team who has been working continually with him this week and so you are the only person who will notice the recurrence of the event.

Rank the actions below in order of most appropriate to least appropriate:

A. Ask the rest of your team if they think your consultant is acting like their normal self today
B. Ask your other junior colleagues in the hospital about the situation
C. Approach the consultant and ask him alone about your concerns
D. Report the consultant to the GMC
E. Accept that the consultant is having a temporary hard time and resolve to interfere if you notice any impact on patient care

Question 98:

You are working as the orthopaedic FY1. Your registrar has asked you to request a CT scan for a patient but you don't know why. You go to speak to the patient about their need for a CT scan and they ask if they can have an MRI scan instead because they are worried about the radiation from a CT scan.

Choose the **THREE** most appropriate actions to take in this situation:

A. Explain the risks and benefits of CT scans, but check the information with official guidelines
B. Call the radiologists to ask about the patient
C. Explain that you are not completely sure why they have had a CT scan ordered but will check with the registrar in question as to why
D. Call the on-call radiologist to have a discussion with the radiologist
E. Tell her that she has been ordered a CT scan for a good reason and she cannot have an MRI scan instead
F. Make a note to ask your registrar the next day about the indications for the CT scan
G. Use this situation as a point for reflection in your ePortfolio so you can be more informed for the future
H. Tell her that MRIs are expensive and only reserved for certain patients

Question 99:

You work closely with another FY1 friend on the ward. One day, they comment that you seem more stressed than usual. You feel embarrassed by this suggestion. You have been feeling very tired, but have attributed this to the stressful nature of the work.

Rank the actions below in order of most appropriate to least appropriate:

A. Ask your friend more about what prompted them to make the comments
B. Ask some other FY1s in the hospital if they think you are stressed
C. Use one of the psychiatric depression screening tools to determine if you should start taking medication to lower your stress
D. Make an appointment with your educational supervisor to discuss that you are stressed
E. Make an appointment with your GP to discuss your concerns

Question 100:

You are part of a small medical team in a district general hospital. You only have one registrar who you've noticed has been turning up to work late regularly which seems out of character. He appears tired and dishevelled. You do not believe patient safety is compromised at this time. You suspect he is abusing alcohol.

Rank the actions below in order of most appropriate to least appropriate:

A. Discuss what you should do with your clinical supervisor in confidence
B. Notify the GMC of your suspicions
C. Escalate your suspicions to their consultant
D. Discuss your opinions with your colleagues
E. Approach the registrar directly but discreetly

Question 101:

You are performing a routine procedure on a patient which you have been judged to be competent to perform. However, there is a routine complication – one which you did not consent them for. The patient wishes to make a formal complaint.

Rank the actions below in order of most appropriate to least appropriate:

F. Notify the consultant in charge of their care
G. Ensure that there are no immediate life-threatening complications
H. Document procedure in the notes
I. Apologise to the patient
J. Offer them information on your local procedures about making a formal complaint

Question 102:

You are asked by a friend who is going on holiday to prescribe him some antibiotics in case he becomes ill.

Rank the actions below in order of most appropriate to least appropriate:

A. Refuse to prescribe him antibiotics
B. Prescribe his antibiotics but only as a private prescription
C. Refuse to prescribe him antibiotics and ask him to go to A&E instead
D. Refuse to prescribe him antibiotics and ask him to go to his GP instead
E. Take a few antibiotic tablets from the drugs trolley and give them to him

Question 103:

You are working as a junior on the gynaecology team. You are the only person of that gender on the team and feel that you are being bullied by the seniors because of it, depriving you of opportunities available to others.

Rank the actions below in order of most appropriate to least appropriate:

A. Organise a meeting and explain directly to your colleagues how you feel and that their behaviour is inappropriate
B. Approach your clinical supervisor about the problem
C. Discuss this with your educational supervisor
D. Send a message saying you are feeling bullied on the group messaging application
E. Notify the foundation programme director that your training is being impaired

Question 104:

You are on call on your birthday and have plans for the evening after your shift. However, the colleague you are handing over to has not arrived. The duty manager informs you they will be at least 30 minutes late.

Rank the actions below in order of most appropriate to least appropriate:

A. Write the jobs on an email and send this to them, then leave
B. Write the handover on a piece of paper and leave it attached to the bleep in the handover room, then leave
C. Leave the bleep and call them later on to give a verbal handover
D. Wait until they arrive to handover
E. Handover to another colleague on that shift and ask them to pass the message on with a written list you have created

Question 105:

You are an FY1 on surgery. You are busy clerking a patient in Accident and Emergency when you are bleeped by nursing staff on the ward. A patient you clerked earlier in the day is in pain. The nurse says that he was transferred to the ward without a drug chart. You distinctly remember writing it and mention this. They then become irate, shout at you and demand that you come and rewrite one immediately.

Rank the actions below in order of most appropriate to least appropriate:

A. Finish clerking your patient
B. Speak to the charge nurse in Accident and Emergency about the incident
C. Go to the ward and rewrite the drug chart
D. Speak to the matron about the nursing staff's behaviour towards you
E. File an incident report regarding loss of the drug chart

Question 106:

You are the FY1 on a particularly understaffed urology team. A patient is about to be discharged home and has been delighted with your care of them. They wish to give some gift vouchers as a thank you.

Rank the actions below in order of most appropriate to least appropriate:

A. Accept the gift and buy presents for the ward staff
B. Ask them to donate the gift to the hospital charitable trust on your behalf
C. Ask them to purchase a communal gift for all the staff on the ward
D. Explain that you cannot accept the gift for professional reasons
E. Thank them for their generous offer

Question 107:

You are working in the community doing paediatrics. A child comes in with their mother with suspicious bruising and behavioural change. The mother is concerned that her partner is becoming violent towards the child. The partner does not live with the mother but usually visits late at night when intoxicated.

Rank the actions below in order of most appropriate to least appropriate:

A. Inform your supervisor
B. Take a full history and examine the child with the mother's consent
C. Inform the designated person for child protection
D. Complete full and detailed documentation of the consultation
E. Inform the police

Question 108:

You are an FY1 on orthopaedic surgery. One of your patients is in a side room and has long-term oxygen therapy at home. He is a lifelong smoker and is three hours post-operation. You can see he is about to light a cigarette.

Rank the actions below in order of most appropriate to least appropriate:

A. Confiscate his lighter
B. Explain to the patient they cannot smoke on hospital premises
C. Ask security to come and assist you
D. Offer him a nicotine patch
E. Let him smoke

Question 109:

You are the FY1 on general surgery in a district general hospital. You are called to see a patient whose family would like to speak to you. The family are upset with the care the patient has received and in particular, that he has been waiting for a magnetic resonance scan for two days. The father becomes aggressive and starts shouting.

Rank the actions below in order of most appropriate to least appropriate:

A. Attempt to de-escalate the situation by apologising to the family
B. Explain why the scan has not happened yet
C. Contact security and ask them to come and assist you
D. Ask a senior to talk to the patient
E. Leave the room

Question 110:

You are an FY1 on the surgical ward. A patient's family friend works as part of the critical care outreach team and is not involved in their care. One day you notice her going through the patient notes and walking in and talking to the patient's family.

Rank the actions below in order of most appropriate to least appropriate:

A. Pull the nurse aside and tell her the behaviour is inappropriate
B. Escalate the problem to the nurse in charge
C. Submit an incident report
D. Notify the information governance team that patient confidentiality has been breached
E. Submit a complaint via PALS

Question 111:

You are the FY1 on the emergency surgical team. You have noticed that a certain registrar seems to be moving all of their shifts to match yours. They also make crude and inappropriate comments which make you feel objectified and uncomfortable.

Rank the actions below in order of most appropriate to least appropriate:

A. Play it off as a joke, and joke back
B. Put up with the comments as your rotation is only two months long
C. Discuss your concerns with them quietly after the ward round
D. Notify the rota coordinator
E. Notify your clinical supervisor

Question 112:

You are the FY1 on weekend medical ward cover. You have been called to see an acutely deteriorating end of life patient and there is no documented escalation plan from their regular team. The medical registrar is too busy and cannot review the patient and has asked you to make decisions regarding their management.

Rank the actions below in order of most appropriate to least appropriate:

A. Stop all their medications
B. Fill out a DNAR form
C. Contact the patient's family
D. Continue resuscitation in the absence of a full plan
E. Contact the out of hours palliative care service

Question 113:

You are allocated to your favourite rotation and want to impress your consultant. They ask you to complete an audit project for them. However, you already have two projects on the go.

Rank the actions below in order of most appropriate to least appropriate:

A. Agree to do the project and give up your off days in order to complete it
B. Kindly decline their offer stating the reason why and offer to ask your colleagues if anyone wants to do it but do not promise anything
C. Kindly decline stating that you have two projects to finish
D. Say you will think about it but do not bring up the subject again
E. Do this project and email your other project supervisors explaining why you will not be completing theirs

Question 114:

You are at a general practice surgery seeing a patient who has recently been diagnosed with epilepsy. Their last seizure was one week ago. They say they are still driving and refuse to give up as it will socially isolate them.

Rank the actions below in order of most appropriate to least appropriate:

A. Explain to the patient that it is imperative that they stop driving
B. State that they have a legal obligation to tell the DVLA that they have epilepsy
C. Explain that if they do not, you will have to notify the DVLA yourself
D. Ask the patients partner to convince them to call the DVLA
E. Inform the DVLA of what is happening

Question 115:

You are at the doctors mess party and you see a colleague who you thought was supposed to be on a night shift. The next day when you return to work, you confirm that they were supposed to be working last night.

Rank the actions below in order of most appropriate to least appropriate:

A. Ask a senior colleague for advice on how to proceed
B. Tell the colleague involved that you won't tell anyone if he works your next on call shift
C. Directly speak to the colleague in question saying that he acted unprofessionally and you will escalate this to management if it happens again
D. Notify your consultant
E. Do nothing

Question 116:

You are in an obstetric outpatient clinic and see a 35-year-old lady from a poor socioeconomic background. The nursing staff report that she admitted to being physically abused at home when she stepped out to provide a urine sample. Her partner is present in the room.

Rank the actions below in order of most appropriate to least appropriate:

A. Ask the partner to leave and discuss with the lady in confidence
B. Approach the subject with the both of them
C. Perform a detailed head to toe examination with a chaperone present
D. Clearly document all the information you have gathered
E. Ask the lady to make a follow up appointment alone

Question 117:

A schizophrenic patient, who is well known to the team, is admitted to hospital with a severe community acquired pneumonia. He is refusing any injections or cannulas. He says, "You are trying to depress my sexual functions with your medications."

Rank the actions below in order of most appropriate to least appropriate:

A. Sedate the patient then cannulate him
B. Ask security personnel to hold him down as you cannulate him
C. Perform a mental capacity assessment
D. Give him oral antibiotics
E. Obey his wishes and do not proceed any further but explain that his life could be in danger without your interventions

Question 118:

You are on weekend ward cover and have been asked to see a frail elderly gentleman who is in pain from metastatic prostate cancer. He calls you over and asks you to end his life by giving him lots of morphine.

Rank the actions below in order of most appropriate to least appropriate:

A. Explore why the patient feels like that
B. Ignore his request
C. Double the morphine prescription dose but not the frequency
D. Call the out of hours palliative care team for advice
E. Ask your registrar for advice

Question 119:

You are consenting a patient for a minor operation that you are comfortable performing. The patient does not speak any English and a translator is present. However, you get the feeling that the translator is not directly paraphrasing what you are saying.

Rank the actions below in order of most appropriate to least appropriate:

A. Ask the patient to sign the consent form
B. Speak to the translator directly and tell them they need to translate word for word
C. Call the translation service and ask them to send you another translator
D. List the patient for the procedure but book another translator on the day of the procedure and sign the consent form then
E. Rebook the outpatient appointment and ask them to bring a family member to translate

Question 120:

You are the surgical FY1. You are called to see a young gentleman who has had multiple admissions under your tenure. He is complaining of nausea but he has not vomited and he is refusing all anti-emetics. He is demanding intravenous cyclizine.

Rank the actions below in order of most appropriate to least appropriate:

A. Prescribe intravenous cyclizine
B. Discuss his rationale for wanting cyclizine
C. Discuss his rationale for refusing other anti-emetics
D. Ask your SHO for advice on what to prescribe
E. Prescribe some intravenous omeprazole and pretend it is cyclizine

Question 121:

You are the FY1 on the diabetes and endocrinology team. You have a 25-year-old gentleman who is a type 1 diabetic and well known for multiple admissions. He is ready for discharge but is homeless. He is refusing to leave and threatening to not take his insulin if he is discharged.

Rank the actions below in order of most appropriate to least appropriate:

A. Discharge the patient regardless
B. Keep the patient in and involve the social services team
C. Explore why the patient does not want to leave as being homeless has not stopped him leaving before
D. Discharge the patient but arrange regular follow up and a point of contact in the diabetic specialist nurse
E. Ask your SHO to see the patient

Question 122:
You are the psychiatry FY2. You walk into the doctor's office and see your colleague drinking wine just prior to the beginning of his shift.

Rank the actions below in order of most appropriate to least appropriate:

A. Throw the bottle away when he leaves and don't say anything
B. Speak to the colleague directly and ask them if they feel they have a problem with alcohol dependence
C. Ask your peers about what you should do if it happens again
D. Ask your peers about what you should do immediately
E. Discuss the issue with your colleague's consultant the next time you see them

Question 123:
It's your first week working as the FY1 in haematology and oncology. A patient is under investigation for suspected acute myeloid leukaemia. They are extremely anxious and are demanding to know their investigation results. You have never met the patient before and you do not know what investigations are normally done for acute myeloid leukaemia.

Rank the actions below in order of most appropriate to least appropriate:

A. Print off the blood results and go through them one by one in an attempt to placate the patient
B. Use an online search engine to find what investigations are done for the condition and how to interpret the results
C. Apologise to the patient and explain that you don't have the expertise to explain the results to him
D. Contact your registrar and ask them to see the patient at their next available opportunity
E. Call the lab to ask what investigations have been ordered and what the results are

Question 124:
A new consultant is doing a medical ward round with you. He prescribes an antibiotic for a patient with a chest infection. You notice that the dose, route and indication are wrong when compared to your hospital guidelines.

Rank the actions below in order of most appropriate to least appropriate:

A. Do nothing – the consultant is probably right
B. Change the antibiotics later on and don't discuss with the consultant
C. Print off the hospital guidelines and show them to the consultant
D. Ask the consultant regarding the rationale for the prescription using it as a teaching opportunity
E. Ask pharmacy for their advice

Question 125:

You are the surgical SHO and your FY1 has asked you to see a patient who is septic postoperatively. You try to contact the registrar but they are performing emergency surgery with the consultant. The operation is in a time critical stage so they cannot be disturbed.

Rank the actions below in order of most appropriate to least appropriate:

A. Contact the critical care outreach team for advice
B. Try to contact the medical registrar for advice
C. Start basic resuscitation treatments
D. Order appropriate investigations
E. Perform an A to E primary assessment

Question 126:

You are the general surgical FY1. The partner of one of your patients approaches you and asks for an update. You have some free time and take her into a quiet room. During the conversation, your patient's partner says, "Thank you for that - you know he didn't even tell me he was having an operation…".

Rank the actions below in order of most appropriate to least appropriate:

A. Document your conversation in the notes
B. Speak to the patient and attempt to gain his consent for discussion with relatives. Then retrospectively document the conversation in the notes
C. Explain to the patient that you have had a discussion with his partner and apologise for not obtaining his consent. Then document both conversations in the notes
D. Document the conversation in the notes stating that you had patient consent
E. Do not document anything

Question 127:

You are the FY1 on general surgery and on a busy surgical take. The surgical registrar is extremely busy. They have just seen a CT report for one of your patients who needs to go to theatre immediately. He asks you to go and consent the patient. What would you do in this scenario?

Rank the actions below in order of most appropriate to least appropriate:

A. Google the common complications then go and consent the patient
B. Go and consent the patient briefly but say that someone else will come back formally to complete the form
C. Ask the surgical registrar if he has jobs for any other patients you can help with and let him consent the patient
D. Explain to the registrar that you cannot consent the patient as an FY1
E. Say that you can book the patient for theatre and speak to the anaesthetist but not consent them

Question 128:

You are part of a busy medical team with an ethos of helping each other out when individuals finish their routine jobs. However, you have consistently noticed that one member at your level does not help out and disappears once their jobs are done. When you raise this issue with them, they reveal that they're sitting an exam and are using the spare time to revise for it.

Rank the actions below in order of most appropriate to least appropriate:

A. Approach your colleague and ask him to help out, saying he should not be using clinical time to revise
B. Escalate the problem to your consultant
C. Inform your colleague's educational supervisor
D. Ask your direct senior to have a word with them
E. Do nothing

Question 129:

A 25-year-old female is admitted to the medical admissions unit with severe alcohol intoxication. She is very aggressive and damaging hospital property.

Rank the actions below in order of most appropriate to least appropriate:

A. Notify the security team
B. Move all other patients out of the way
C. Try to talk the patient down
D. Sedate the patient
E. Ask other team members to assist you in physically restraining the patient

Question 130:

A young patient has been in hospital for 4 weeks on the endocrine ward and you have become quite friendly with them. On discharge, they thank you and give you wine and chocolates. When you get home that day you notice that they have added you as a friend on a social media platform.

Rank the actions below in order of most appropriate to least appropriate:

A. Ask for the advice of your colleagues at the next MDT meeting
B. Send them a letter saying why you cannot add them
C. Add them
D. Do not add them or respond
E. Send them a message saying thank you but that you do not add patients on social media

Question 131:
It is lunchtime and you head to the local market to grab some food. When you return, you notice that your list is missing and are suspicious that you have left it at the food stall. The list is not at the food stall when you go back to check.

Rank the actions below in order of most appropriate to least appropriate:

A. Print off a new list and use that instead
B. Submit an incident report
C. Notify your colleagues that you have lost your list
D. Take a colleague's list and pretend it is yours
E. Find your consultant and ask for their advice

Question 132:
You are called to the ward to see a patient. Your registrar has spoken to the family and broken the diagnosis of metastatic prostate cancer. However, they did not tell the patient who is now very upset that he's found out via his family and not directly from the medical team.

Rank the actions below in order of most appropriate to least appropriate:

A. Apologise to the patient
B. Break the bad news to the patient
C. Inform your registrar about the miscommunication
D. Ask your registrar to come and break the bad news to the patient
E. Submit an incident report

Question 133:
You see a 70-year-old lady in clinic who has advanced pancreatic cancer. After hearing the benefits and drawbacks of palliative chemotherapy she politely declines further treatment as she doesn't feel up to it. Her partner says that she is being silly and that you should ignore her.

Rank the actions below in order of most appropriate to least appropriate:

A. Explain that every patient has the right to refuse treatment
B. Say that you try to take the opinions of the family into consideration in certain scenarios
C. Document the consultation clearly in the notes
D. Ignore the patient's request as you see they have a diagnosis of dementia in their past medical history
E. Empathise with the partner by saying that this is a very difficult decision to make

Question 134:
You are working on a night shift as the surgical FY1. You walk into the doctor's mess and see that the paediatric registrar is watching child pornography. He turns around and notices you.

Rank the actions below in order of most appropriate to least appropriate:

A. Pretend you didn't see anything and leave
B. Directly confront the registrar
C. Report him to the consultant on call
D. Speak to the site practitioners
E. Inform the GMC

Question 135:
You are the orthopaedic SHO and are reviewing an eight-year-old child. They are bleeding profusely from a leg wound after a car versus bicycle accident. The mother tells you that they are a Jehovah's Witness and do not want him to have blood. The team, including the consultant, agree that he needs an urgent blood transfusion.

Rank the actions below in order of most appropriate to least appropriate:

A. Treat the child in their best interests and give them blood
B. Begin aggressive fluid resuscitation
C. Ask the child what they want
D. Contact the legal team
E. Do not give the child any blood products

Question 136:
You are seeing a 50-year-old lady in your GP clinic. She is run down, thin and gaunt. She is unkempt and is not looking after herself. She admits that she doesn't cook or wash as she doesn't have the energy. She has the clinical features of severe depression.

Rank the actions below in order of most appropriate to least appropriate:

A. Screen for suicidal ideation
B. Inform your senior GP partner
C. Inform social services
D. Ask for a rapid psychiatric assessment
E. Start her on antidepressant medication

Question 137:

A 13-year-old girl attends your GP clinic. She admits to being sexually active with another 13-year-old and is requesting contraception.

Rank the actions below in order of most appropriate to least appropriate:

A. Write a prescription for contraception as you assume she is "Gillick" competent
B. Assess to see how much she knows about contraception
C. Explain the benefits and drawbacks of contraception
D. Ask her to repeat the information back to you
E. Ask her to rebook an appointment with her mother

Question 138:

You are a FY2 working in A&E. An 83-year-old man with dementia is brought to the emergency department after falling down the stairs. You suspect he has a severe fracture of his pelvis and is bleeding profusely from it. He is confused and agitated, but you are unable to determine what his normal level of function is. You determine that he lacks capacity.

Rank the actions below in order of most appropriate to least appropriate:

A. Begin aggressive resuscitation
B. Ask for an urgent surgical review from the orthopaedic registrar with a view to listing them for theatre
C. Contact the next of kin to establish a baseline function
D. Start the patient on end-of-life palliative medications
E. Fill in a Do Not Attempt Cardiopulmonary Resuscitation (DNACPR) order

Question 139:

You are the FY1 working a quiet Saturday shift. Your consultant calls you directly and asks you to go and see one of his patients on the private ward who has become unstable.

Rank the actions below in order of most appropriate to least appropriate:

A. Ask the consultant to call your SHO for the review
B. Check with your medico-legal provider
C. Decline their request stating FY1s are not allowed to see private patients
D. Ask for compensation for services rendered
E. Agree to go and see the patient

Question 140:

You are the gastroenterology FY2. One of your patients is extremely angry that he has not had his colonoscopy in the past 2 days due to "emergencies." He wants to go privately and is asking you to call the private hospital on his behalf to arrange transfer.

Rank the actions below in order of most appropriate to least appropriate:

A. Ask your clinical supervisor on how to proceed
B. Refuse his request stating you do not have any obligation to arrange his transfer
C. Ask one of the consultants to come and see him about going privately
D. Call endoscopy and try to get a date and time for his colonoscopy
E. Give the patient the contact details of the hospital and ask him to arrange transfer

Question 141:

A patient is admitted under your ENT team with tonsillitis. Her blood tests show that she is HIV positive. She was neither consented nor counselled prior to this test being done.

Rank the actions below in order of most appropriate to least appropriate:

A. Refer the patient to the GUM team for follow up
B. Explain what the plan is from here and the treatment options
C. Take a full sexual history
D. Break the news to the patient
E. Explain to the patient what blood test results were taken and the rationale behind them

Question 142:

A surgical registrar obtained a needle stick injury in theatre. Blood tests were done and the Hepatitis C serology results have come back positive. The registrar has explicitly told you not to tell anyone the results. The next week you see them still performing exposure prone procedures.

Rank the actions below in order of most appropriate to least appropriate:

A. Escalate to the regional surgical education programme director
B. Notify the consultant of the test results
C. Notify occupational health of the result
D. Pull them to one side and ask them if they have informed occupational health
E. Notify the GMC

Question 143:

You are completing a discharge summary for one of your patients who has known breast cancer. They have had a CT scan today which shows metastatic breast cancer. The patient's daughter calls you and asks about their progress and CT scan results.

Rank the actions below in order of most appropriate to least appropriate:

A. Explain that they are ready for discharge
B. Explain that the CT scan showed progression of the malignancy
C. Go and ask the patient if it is okay to update their daughter
D. Pass the phone to the nursing staff and ask them to update the family
E. Say you cannot update them at this time over the phone as you have not given the results to the patient yet

Question 144:

You are an FY2 and covering medical wards with another FY1 doctor. You have previously not got on well with them as they tended talk down to you and bully you. The registrar has not turned up. They FY1 doctor feels very confident and decides to take the bleep and starts to issue orders.

Rank the actions below in order of most appropriate to least appropriate:

A. Take the bleep yourself until the registrar arrives
B. Leave the handover room and ignore all of the FY1's orders
C. Contact the site practitioners to notify them the registrar has not arrived
D. Explain that they do not have the experience to hold the registrar bleep
E. Explain that they are less experienced than you and they have no right to issue orders

Question 145:

You are on a busy ENT team with two FY2s. You notice that they leave promptly after the ward round and do not help out with the jobs but go to theatre. All three of you are considering ENT as a career.

Rank the actions below in order of most appropriate to least appropriate:

A. Put an angry message on the group messaging application
B. Ask the registrars to have a word with the team members
C. Discuss with your clinical supervisor that you are being deprived of opportunities
D. Post a rant on a social network clearly naming the involved colleagues
E. Explain to your educational supervisor that you are being deprived of opportunities

Question 146:
You are one of three upper gastrointestinal surgery FY1s at a district general hospital. You find that you have a very light workload with minimal learning opportunities. You and your colleagues do not feel your educational experience is adequate.

Rank the actions below in order of most appropriate to least appropriate:

A. Fill your spare time with audit and quality improvement projects
B. Help out the colorectal team who tend to be inundated with jobs and patients daily
C. Raise the unequal distribution of workload with the foundation programme director
D. Study for an exam
E. Hone your pool skills in the doctors' mess

Question 147:
A patient on the gastroenterology ward is detoxing from alcohol dependence. They are being verbally aggressive to staff. A nurse comes to you and is very clearly upset with the situation.

Rank the actions below in order of most appropriate to least appropriate:

A. Ask her to speak to the matron about the patient
B. Advise the nurse to ignore that patient
C. Suggest the nurse changes bays to avoid the patient
D. Ask the patient to apologise to the nurse
E. Tell the nurse you will go and speak to the patient

Question 148:
A very difficult patient has been admitted under your emergency surgical team. She is known to be very manipulative and has successfully sued the trust on three previous occasions. She has five abdominal operations because she always demands one for her abdominal pain.

Rank the actions below in order of most appropriate to least appropriate:

A. List the patient for another operation should she request it
B. Seek advice from the legal team at the hospital
C. Only see the patient in groups with appropriate chaperones
D. Be meticulous with your documentation
E. Do not see the patient on your ward rounds

Question 149:

You are in a GP practice. One of your regular patients who is HIV positive comes to see you. You ask about their recent sexual history and they disclose that they have a new partner but are not using barrier protection. Your patient refuses to engage with treatment under the GUM team due to the side effects. They have not told their partner of their HIV status.

Rank the actions below in order of most appropriate to least appropriate:

A. Try to convince the patient to tell their partner
B. State that you have a responsibility to notify their partner
C. Offer to arrange an appointment for them together
D. Attempt to convince the patient to use barrier contraception
E. Do not disclose any information as it breaches confidentiality

Question 150:

You are the urology FY1. A nurse wants some personal advice regarding her urinary symptoms. She asks you to write her a prescription for some antibiotics.

Rank the actions below in order of most appropriate to least appropriate:

A. Ask her to go to Accident and Emergency so you can prescribe it
B. Say that she should just take some from the drug trolley
C. Ask her to see her GP
D. Prescribe antibiotics on a private prescription form
E. Refuse to give advice

Question 151:

You are finishing your on call day shift. You are asked to prescribe warfarin so it can be given at the normal time. However, when you check, the latest INR blood result is not back from the lab.

Rank the actions below in order of most appropriate to least appropriate:

A. Prescribe the same warfarin dose as yesterday
B. Call the lab to try and find out the results
C. Hand over the job to the night team
D. Explain to the nurses that you cannot dose the warfarin without the INR
E. Ignore the request as it is the end of your shift

Question 152:
You are the haematology FY1 and are asked to cannulate a patient for their antibiotics. You have been unsuccessful four times on the same patient before. The patient recognises you and refuses to let you cannulate them.

Rank the actions below in order of most appropriate to least appropriate:

A. Proceed with cannulation saying that it is in the best interests of the patient
B. Perform a mental capacity assessment
C. Call the anaesthetic team for help as this patient is very difficult to cannulate
D. Ask your SHO to come and cannulate the patient
E. Walk away documenting in the notes that the patient refused

Question 153:
You have an FY1 colleague who has been turning up late to work for several weeks. Tonight, she turns up to her night shift in tears and walks out of handover.

Choose the **THREE** most appropriate options.

A. Write a list of jobs for her and text her where you have left them
B. Sit down and talk about her problems
C. Notify your mutual clinical supervisor
D. Suggests she takes sick leave
E. Notify the site practitioners that she is not fit to work
F. Advise her to speak to her educational supervisor
G. Seek advice from your educational supervisor
H. Advise her to see her GP

Question 154:
A 14-year-old boy comes to Accident and Emergency with his friends after falling off his bicycle whilst doing stunts on a ramp. He smells heavily of alcohol and admits to drinking vodka in the park. He does not want you to call his parents. He wants some painkillers but no other treatment. Radiographs show a greenstick fracture of the ulna.

Choose the **THREE** most appropriate options.

A. Contact his GP surgery to notify them what has happened
B. Call his parents yourself without letting him know
C. Prescribe painkillers and let him go
D. Try to convince him to call his parents and let them know what has happened
E. Refer to the paediatrics team for further advice on how to manage the situation
F. Ask his friends to convince him to have the appropriate treatment
G. Notify social services
H. Refuse to let him self-discharge until treated fully for the fracture

Question 155:

You are in a general paediatric clinic. You see a 14-year-old boy who is short and is being bullied at school. His parents ask if he could have growth hormone treatment. However, when plotting his growth chart, you see he is at the mid-parental height.

Choose the **THREE** most appropriate options.

A. Explain your findings on the growth chart to the family
B. Explore the parent's reasons for wanting growth hormone
C. Contact the child's school to notify them about the bullying
D. Ask the child his thoughts about undergoing treatment
E. Explain the advantages + disadvantages of undergoing growth hormone therapy
F. Check your prescription is correct with the senior GP
G. Refuse to prescribe the growth hormone therapy
H. Tell them about the disadvantages of using growth hormone therapy

Question 156:

A 30-year-old woman self-presented to A&E after taking a paracetamol overdose. She does not wish to disclose how many tablets or over what time period she took them. She is refusing any treatment and says that she wants to die. She understands that refusing treatment may cause her to die.

Choose the **THREE** most appropriate options.

A. Seek advice from the medico-legal team about how to proceed
B. Treat her under the mental health act
C. Treat her under the mental capacity act
D. Arrange an urgent psychiatric assessment
E. Ask for a senior review
F. Discharge her if she is refusing any treatment
G. Ask security for assistance whilst you cannulate and treat her
H. Respect her right to refuse treatment

Question 157:

A 35-year-old is brought into A&E after a major road traffic collision. You have a high clinical suspicion that they have severe intra-abdominal bleeding which is confirmed on ultrasound. Haemodynamically they are in extremis. They state they are a Jehovah's Witness and are refusing a blood transfusion.

Choose the **THREE** most appropriate options.

A. Arrange a crossmatch urgently
B. Call their relatives and ask them to convince the patient to change their mind
C. Transfuse them as you feel it is in their best interests
D. Perform a mental capacity assessment
E. Speak to the legal team
F. Respect their decision to refuse transfusion
G. Consult your local guidelines on the use of auto-transfusion
H. Explain that refusing a transfusion is potentially life threatening

Question 158:

You are the FY2 on general surgery. You have been asked to consent a patient with suspected appendicitis for an appendectomy. You know some, but not all of the complications of the procedure.

Choose the **THREE** most appropriate options.

A. Consent for the complications you know
B. Refuse to consent the patient as you are not comfortable doing it
C. Ask the registrar to consent the patient
D. Explain the procedure to the patient
E. Explain the need for the procedure to the patient
F. Fill the consent form and ask the patient to sign but do not sign it yourself
G. Ask them to sign the consent form but fill in the complications later after discussion with your registrar

Question 159:

A senior colleague approaches you at the end of the ward round; they feel you are slow and not picking up your fair share of the routine jobs. They say that if you do not improve, they will escalate to the consultant.

Choose the **THREE** most appropriate options.

A. Ignore them, you know you are doing your fair share
B. Ask them to explain their reasoning
C. Ask your educational supervisor for advice
D. Ask your colleagues if they feel the same about you
E. Agree with them and then do not change anything
F. Escalate to your consultant saying you feel bullied
G. Make an action plan to show how you plan to improve
H. Explain to them this is your first job and you are bound to be slow

Question 160:

You are part of a four-man junior doctor endocrine team which is split in pairs between two consultants. You have noticed that the two doctors on the other team are not getting along. The more senior colleague is publicly shouting at and embarrassing the junior colleague in front of patients, families and other staff.

Choose the **THREE** most appropriate options.

A. Speak to your clinical supervisor about the matter
B. Sit down as a group and maturely discuss the problems
C. Change teams so the other two are split up
D. Sit with your junior colleague on the other team and explore how they feel about the situation
E. Recommend that they escalate to their clinical supervisor
F. Ignore the situation, it is not affecting your half of the team
G. Notify the foundation programme director
H. Notify the medical education department

Question 161:

A patient calls you over to their bedside. They say that their iPad has been stolen.

Choose the **THREE** most appropriate options.

A. Notify the security personnel
B. Notify the police
C. Help search the patient's belongings
D. Ask the patient to submit a PALS complaint
E. Search all the other patients' belongings in that bay
F. Dismiss the case because the patient has dementia
G. Send an email to all the ward staff notifying of the theft
H. Pass the information on to the ward sister

Question 162:

You are the FY2 on obstetrics and gynaecology. A conversation is taking place between a midwife and the consultant. The consultant is being rude to the midwife and is acting superior. When the consultant leaves, you overhear the midwife talking to the other midwives about his behaviour, how it happens frequently, and makes the midwives feel uncomfortable.

Choose the **THREE** most appropriate options.

A. Do nothing and let the midwives sort it out
B. Ask the patients how they feel about the behaviour
C. Ask your clinical supervisor on how to proceed
D. Discuss how often this is happening with midwives
E. Speak to the consultant directly
F. Notify the head midwife
G. Notify the matron of obstetrics and gynaecology
H. Apologise on behalf of the consultant

Question 163:

You are the medical FY2 on the acute medical admissions unit. You happen to live in the doctors' accommodation with your registrar. They are extremely messy and leave dishes and food lying around in the kitchen at home. You have had an argument about it and it is now affecting your working relationship.

Choose the **THREE** most appropriate options.

A. Ask them to be cleaner at home and then explain that you won't have a problem at work
B. Notify your consultant that your working relationship is impaired
C. It is not affecting patient safety so you do not need to do anything
D. Ask the foundation programme director to move you to a different rotation
E. Sit down with the registrar and try to work out your differences
F. Ask other colleagues to see if they think your professionalism is being impaired
G. Ask your patient's if they believe your professionalism is being impaired
H. Notify your educational supervisor

Question 164:

You are the FY1 on general surgery and are finishing a ward round. You and your core trainee walk out of a room where you have had a difficult conversation with a patient. The core trainee uses a derogatory racial slur to describe the patient. You are unsure as to whether the patient heard this.

Choose the **THREE** most appropriate options.

A. Do nothing as it is an isolated incident
B. Agree with the core trainee
C. Say nothing, but document in the notes that they have used that language
D. Approach the core trainee and say that their language was inappropriate
E. Notify the ward sister
F. Submit an incident form
G. Notify your clinical supervisor that this has happened

Question 165:

You are the FY1 on trauma and orthopaedics. You attended the doctor's mess party last night and noticed that your FY2 drank lots of alcohol. They have not turned up for work as they have called in sick. You have been forced to cover their on call.

Choose the **THREE** **least** appropriate options.

A. Notify your consultant as to the real reason they are not at work
B. Send an angry message to your FY2
C. Send a message to your FY2 saying that you will cover their on call but they must do two of yours in return
D. Notify occupational health that you believe your colleague has an alcohol dependency problem
E. Email the department highlighting the issue that the FY2 continually does this
F. Notify the foundation programme director
G. Notify the medical education department

Question 166:

You are late to work because your alarm did not go off. You cannot function without having breakfast. You collapsed on the ward round the last time that tried to work without breakfast. You know the team will be waiting for you to do the ward round.

Choose the **THREE** most appropriate options.

A. Have breakfast and accept that you are already late
B. Call the team and apologise. Stop at the coffee shop on the way in
C. Offer to buy everybody coffee as an excuse
D. Go straight to ward round, everybody is waiting
E. Call in sick as you will be too embarrassed
F. Call the consultant directly and apologise, have breakfast then go to work
G. Call the team and say your car has broken down

Question 167:

You and your colorectal colleagues have been asked by the director of surgery to complete the morbidity and mortality presentation for the next meeting. When you try and start, all your colleagues say that they are busy and refuse to help you.

Choose the **THREE** most appropriate options.

A. Do the presentation alone
B. Refuse to do the presentation without help because it is too much work
C. Email the director of surgery and notify them of your problem
D. Send a message on the group messaging application which includes your registrars to ask for help
E. Notify the foundation programme director
F. Ask your clinical supervisor for advice on how to complete the presentation alone
G. Do some of the presentation proportional to your fair share and then tell your colleagues that it is their responsibility to complete it
H. Say to the others that they can do all the ward work whilst you complete the morbidity and mortality presentation

Question 168:

You are the medical FY1 on intensive care. You notice that a core trainee is going into the controlled drugs cupboard and taking fentanyl vials and putting them in his bag.

Choose the **THREE** most appropriate options.

A. Notify the GMC
B. Notify your consultant of your suspicions
C. Notify the chief pharmacist that it appears some controlled drugs are unaccounted for
D. Note in the controlled drugs book that he has taken fentanyl from the cupboard to keep a record of it
E. Secretly take the fentanyl out of his bag and replace it in the cupboard
F. Ask your colleagues if they have noticed any similar behaviour from the core trainee in question
G. Notify the matron of intensive care of your suspicions
H. Approach the trainee directly and ask about illicit drug use

Question 169:

You are the FY1 on general surgery. Your registrar has asked you to do their teaching session for the medical students tomorrow as they do not have time. The session is on interpreting abdominal radiological investigations – a topic which you are not wholly confident with.

Choose the **THREE** most appropriate options.

A. Refuse to do the session by being open and honest with the registrar and stating that you do not feel qualified to give the session
B. Ask a radiology registrar to cover for the surgical registrar
C. Give the session but change the content to a general surgical topic you are comfortable with
D. Cancel the teaching session and rearrange it
E. Ask your consultant if they would be able to give the session instead
F. Ask if there is an available core surgical trainee to give the session
G. Use a search engine to find a presentation and just read off the slides
H. Do some reading to improve your knowledge and prepare a presentation for the next day

Question 170:

You are on a consultant ward round with the respiratory team. You feel that the consultant is ordering inappropriate and unnecessary investigations which may be harming patients.

Choose the **THREE** most appropriate options.

A. Ask the consultant each time to justify his choice of investigations and document it
B. Document the plans and that you feel the investigations may be unnecessary
C. Do not order the investigations
D. Explain the risks and benefits of each investigation to patients and then ask if they want them
E. Ask your clinical supervisor about how to proceed
F. Submit an incident form
G. Order the investigations because they are ultimately in charge of the patient
H. Ask another consultant to review the patients after this ward round has finished

Question 171:

You are the supernumerary FY1 on paediatrics. For the last few weeks, you feel that you are not learning very much. Since you are unable to perform procedures, you are not meeting your ePortfolio requirements.

Choose the **THREE** most appropriate options.

A. Contact the foundation programme director
B. Spend most of your time helping out other specialties in order to achieve your competencies
C. Arrange a meeting with your educational supervisor to make a plan
D. Discuss the problem with your clinical supervisor
E. Ask the SHOs to fill out forms to make it look like you are achieving your competencies
F. Reflect upon the lack of opportunities
G. Ask the consultants to give you a clinic room in which you can see patients during their clinics
H. Do not worry about it as you will be able to make it back up in the next two rotations

Question 172:

Your hospital has very strict infection control procedures because of several recent outbreaks of *Norovirus* and *Clostridium difficile*. During a hand hygiene audit, your department has come up as the worst in the hospital.

Choose the **THREE** most appropriate options.

A. List this as a point of discussion at the next morbidity and mortality meeting
B. Inform the consultant director of the department
C. Ask them to repeat the audit stating that it was unfair that they were not notified
D. Ensure your personal hand hygiene practices are up to standard
E. Raise the issue at every ward round, before and after seeing every patient
F. It is not your concern - let more senior members deal with the issue
G. Audit it yourself as you do not believe the figures.

Question 173:

You are approached by a consultant geriatrician. They state that your clothing and attire over the past week has been inappropriate. They have told you to go home and change clothes.

Choose the **THREE** most appropriate options.

A. Ask your clinical supervisor for advice
B. Send an email to the geriatric consultant asking them to explain what they think you need to change
C. Go home and change
D. Go and change into scrubs for the day
E. Go shopping and change all of your outfits
F. Ask your colleagues if they think your attire is unprofessional
G. Ignore the allegation and do nothing
H. Submit a complaint citing workplace bullying

Question 174:

You are hoping to study for the MRCP in order to take it this coming January. It is a pre-requisite to getting a competitive training post that you have been gearing yourself up for the past 2 years. However, your rota is missing two doctors and you have to pick up the extra workload.

Choose the **THREE** most appropriate options.

A. Refuse to do the on call shifts
B. Notify the department that they should arrange for locum cover for the unfilled shifts
C. Cover the shifts as patient safety is at risk
D. Arrange a meeting with your educational supervisor
E. Postpone the exam
F. Aim to sit the exam anyway and prepare as best as you can
G. Discuss the problem with your clinical supervisor

Question 175:

You are the acute medicine FY1. You have arranged for one of your patients to have a blood transfusion. Just before you leave for the evening, the lab call you to say the blood is ready. However, you forgot to hand this over to the FY1 on call overnight and to the nursing staff.

Rank the actions below in order of most appropriate to least appropriate:

A. Contact the FY1 who you handed over to and notify them
B. Tell the staff the next day as it can wait overnight
C. Go back and hand over in person
D. Call the ward and notify the nurse in charge
E. Call the on call registrar and ask them to pass the message on

Question 176:

You are on a twilight evening shift and have just seen a patient who needs antibiotics for a severe bone infection. The patient is allergic to the first-line antibiotic and you do not know what the next most appropriate antibiotic would be.

Rank the actions below in order of most appropriate to least appropriate:

A. Call the on call pharmacist and ask what to use
B. Call the microbiology consultant on call for advice
C. Search the BNF for what to prescribe
D. Search the hospital intranet for guidelines on what to prescribe
E. Ask your registrar what to prescribe

Question 177:

You are working a busy Saturday shift but have been feeling unwell for the past few hours. You suspect you have food poisoning from a take-away meal that you reheated yesterday. You develop nausea and vomiting at 3PM.

Rank the actions below in order of most appropriate to least appropriate:

A. Stay as it is a busy ward and you feel bad for handing over the jobs to the on call SHO
B. Take an anti-emetic from the drug trolley and continue
C. Inform the on call registrar
D. Hand over your jobs to the SHO, then go home
E. Complete your urgent jobs and then leave

Question 178:

You have a patient with progressive motor neurone disease. He has got to a stage where he is unable to communicate verbally or with writing but relies on eye movements. You notice in his notes that he has previously arranged an advanced directive about his care but this is not currently available. You ask him if he wants a DNAR and he signals that he does. However, he is unable to sign the form and has no next of kin.

Rank the actions below in order of most appropriate to least appropriate:

A. Sign the DNAR form, it seems like the patient wants it
B. Seek legal advice regarding the advanced directive
C. Do not fill a form in as you cannot be sure that the patient wants this
D. Ask your registrar to complete the DNAR form
E. Contact the patient's lawyer to retrieve a copy of the advanced directive

Question 179:

You are the surgical FY1 on the Hepatobilliary team. One of your patients has had a liver resection for metastasis of colorectal cancer. You have noticed that their LFTs are significantly deranged so you review and alter their medications appropriately. The next day you notice the nursing staff are giving the old doses to that patient.

Rank the actions below in order of most appropriate to least appropriate:

A. Ask the nurses why the wrong doses are being given
B. Complete an incident report
C. Document your discussion in the notes
D. Notify the ward sister of what has happened
E. Apologise to the patient

Question 180:

It is coming towards the end of your first FY1 rotation. You have been struggling to arrange a meeting with your clinical supervisor as they have cancelled on each occasion. You are worried that you may fail the rotation if this is not completed on your ePortfolio on time.

Rank the actions below in order of most appropriate to least appropriate:

A. Ask the secretary to put another date in the respective consultant's diary
B. Send an email to the foundation programme director about the situation
C. Notify your local medical education department
D. Ask a different consultant to fill in the ePortfolio form
E. Fill the form in yourself

Question 181:

You are on the orthopaedic ward and walk past a patient's bedside. You notice the nursing staff are being rather rough with a patient. When they are finished you approach them about their behaviour. They say that the patient is demented and they had to be rough with them.

Rank the actions below in order of most appropriate to least appropriate:

A. Fill in an incident report
B. Apologise to the patient
C. Notify the matron of the ward
D. Do nothing as it is not your patient
E. Document what you saw and the conversation in the notes

Question 182:

You are the FY1 on general surgery. You have a well-liked, long-term inpatient with a high output stoma and significant kidney injury. However, they also have significant heart failure and have had two intensive care admissions with fluid overload. You are limiting their intravenous fluid therapy very carefully for this reason to five hundred millilitres every 24 hours. When you return to work one morning you notice the patient has one litre running. There is no fluid prescription on the drug chart but the nurses said the patient's mouth felt dry so they started more fluid because they felt sorry for her. They ask you to prescribe it "in retrospect".

Rank the actions below in order of most appropriate to least appropriate:

A. Prescribe the fluid because it is your patient and it has now been given
B. Refuse to sign the prescription
C. Notify your consultant
D. Escalate to the ward sister
E. Fill in an incident report

Question 183:

You are on your final FY1 rotation - elective orthopaedics. You have a peculiar patient that keeps getting visits late in the evenings from different female friends. One evening when you walk past their side room, you notice illicit sexual activity happening.

Rank the actions below in order of most appropriate to least appropriate:

A. Knock on the door giving them time to stop before entering
B. Call security
C. Pretend nothing happened
D. Document the events in the notes
E. Notify the ward staff of what has been happening

Question 184:

You have been dating one of your FY1 colleagues for 6 months now. However, it is coming to the end of the year and you are both moving on to new trusts that are extremely distant to each other. You decide to end the relationship but feel now the awkwardness is affecting your work and social life.

Rank the actions below in order of most appropriate to least appropriate:

A. Discuss with other colleagues about how to proceed
B. Discuss with the other FY1 you were in a relationship with on how they feel
C. Discuss the problem with your educational supervisor
D. Avoid your colleague
E. Don't do anything, it is the end of the year soon

Question 185:

You are called to see an acutely delirious patient overnight on a geriatrics ward. They are incredibly aggressive and have already injured one member of staff. They are at risk of harming other patients and not responding to any attempts to calm them down.

Rank the actions below in order of most appropriate to least appropriate:

A. Call security
B. Sedate the patient pharmacologically
C. Try to calm them down by sitting and talking to them
D. Ask security to forcibly restrain the patient
E. Ask other staff members to forcibly restrain the patient

Question 186:

You are studying in a university library. You notice that some medical students seem to have a copy of the upcoming neurology exam paper and are discussing potential answers amongst themselves.

Rank the actions below in order of most appropriate to least appropriate:

A. Send an email to the medical school about your suspicions that some students seem to have the exam paper but do not name anyone
B. Tell the students that you will be reporting them
C. Covertly take their names down and report them
D. Help them with the paper as it is good revision for you as well
E. Do nothing as you are not involved in teaching therefore it is not your problem

Question 187:

You are with your registrars at the Christmas mess party. You walk into the toilet and see one of them snorting a line of cocaine. You leave before they see you.

Rank the actions below in order of most appropriate to least appropriate:

A. Pretend that the event did not occur
B. Send an email to your consultant notifying them about the event
C. Discuss with the other registrars to see if they have noticed similar behaviour
D. Speak to the offending registrar and try to ascertain how often they use illicit substances
E. Monitor the situation to see if it is occurring more often and impacting upon their clinical acumen

Question 188:

Junior doctors on most medical wards get consultant-led bedside teaching once per week. However, on your cardiology firm they do not. You feel you are missing out on an important educational opportunity to prepare for your membership exams.

Rank the actions below in order of most appropriate to least appropriate:

A. Go to the teaching on other firms
B. Notify the medical education department
C. Discuss the issues at the next audit meeting with the consultants
D. Organise a teaching programme from the registrars
E. Find the patients others are seeing and go and see them yourself

Question 189:

You are the FY2 on diabetes and endocrinology. You are in clinic with one of the consultants. He asks you to start seeing patients on your own. However, you do not feel you should be seeing patients alone due to your clinical inexperience.

Rank the actions below in order of most appropriate to least appropriate:

A. See the patients alone - you know where the consultant will be if you need advice
B. Ask the nurses to only schedule you one or two patients at first
C. Deliberately take a long time so you only see the minimal amounts of patients during clinic
D. Agree but then say you have been called away to the ward
E. Agree to see patients but say you will need to run every management plan by them

Question 190:

You are the respiratory FY1 and seeing a respiratory patient on a surgical ward as they are an 'outlier'. A nurse asks you to rewrite a drug chart for one of the surgical patients. It is 3PM and you are still on your ward round.

Rank the actions below in order of most appropriate to least appropriate:

A. Take the drug chart and say you will write it but then continue on your ward round
B. Prescribe the one medication they want to give and leave the rest
C. Rewrite the drug chart as it will get them off your back
D. Ask them to call the surgical team
E. Refuse to rewrite the drug chart

Question 191:

You are the FY1 on gastroenterology. You have dyed your hair pink for a breast cancer charity run. A patient's relative approaches you and says that you look unprofessional. They submit an official complaint and do not want you involved with the patient's care anymore.

Rank the actions below in order of most appropriate to least appropriate:

A. Refuse to acknowledge the complaint and continue to treat the patient
B. Apologise to the patient and attempt to convince them to allow you to continue to participate in their care
C. Do not participate in the patient's care
D. Only participate in their care from afar covertly, but do not go into the room at any time
E. Apologise to the family via a letter

Question 192:

You are the FY1 on acute assessment unit (AAU). It was a religious festival last week and you are wearing wrist apparel from it. You are called aside by the infection control nurse who tells you that you are breaking the trust "bare below the elbow" policy.

Rank the actions below in order of most appropriate to least appropriate:

A. Ask your colleagues what you should do
B. Refuse to acknowledge their warning
C. Acknowledge their warning but do not change your practice
D. Remove the wrist apparel
E. Say that this is religious apparel and they cannot force you to take it off as it would be discriminatory

Question 193:
You are the orthopaedics FY1. You are a keen cyclist but suffered an ankle injury after a collision on the weekend. Your ward rounds are extremely fast paced and you are concerned that you will not be able to keep up. The last time you were slow on the ward round, the consultant continually shouted at you and embarrassed you in front of patients.

Rank the actions below in order of most appropriate to least appropriate:

A. Call in sick until you are able to walk at full pace
B. Notify occupational health of your concerns
C. Email your consultant before the ward round and explain your concerns
D. Switch teams that week so you can avoid the consultant
E. Bear with it and go to work as normal

Question 194:
You are one of two FY1s on the cardiology team. You are concerned that your colleague is depressed as their mood has changed significantly since starting the job and they do not seem to be eating or engaging with anyone like they were. It is not currently having an impact on patient care as you are picking up the slack.

Rank the actions below in order of most appropriate to least appropriate:

A. Notify their clinical supervisor of your concerns
B. Notify your educational supervisor of your concerns
C. Take some time out and sit with your fellow FY1 to explore the problem
D. Do nothing as it is not your place to interfere
E. Speak to your colleagues to see if they have noticed similar changes

Question 195:
You are one of three FY2s on the medical oncology team. Each FY2 is scheduled to go to monthly teaching on a certain Thursday each month. However, one month you have a problem with this as one colleague is on nights and the other has booked annual leave. If you go, this will leave the ward unattended.

Rank the actions below in order of most appropriate to least appropriate:

A. Do not attend teaching as being on the ward is more important
B. Tell your FY2 colleague that they cannot take their annual leave as you need to go to teaching
C. Notify your educational supervisor of the problem
D. Try to rearrange your teaching and go at a different time
E. Ask a friend to sign you in to teaching

Question 196:
You are a hardworking member of the ENT team. You have submitted a paper which has been accepted for presentation at an international conference. However, the registrar has said that they will present it despite you having done all of the work.

Rank the actions below in order of most appropriate to least appropriate:

A. Refuse to provide them with any of your work
B. Let them present it but ensure your name is on it
C. Report them to the GMC
D. Notify your supervising consultant
E. Create a false set of results and send those to them. Then work on the real results

Question 197:
You are the general surgery FY1. You need to get catheterisation signed-off to complete your ePortfolio. You know the urology FY1 has plenty of catheterisations to do each week. You ask them multiple times to let you know when there is a patient that needs catheterising. However, they never tell you when there are some to do.

Rank the actions below in order of most appropriate to least appropriate:

A. Notify their clinical supervisor about their behaviour
B. Try to find a different specialty that has catheters for you to do
C. Ask the urology SHO when they have catheters that need doing
D. Tell your educational supervisor about your difficulties in finding catheters
E. Catheterise one of your patients for the experience

Question 198:
You are the medical student teaching programme co-ordinator. The teaching is compulsory for the students but three of them consistently do not turn up.

Rank the actions below in order of most appropriate to least appropriate:

A. Do nothing - assume someone in the medical education team will look into it
B. Report them to the medical education team locally
C. Ask to meet the three students in a group and discuss the reasons as to why they are not attending
D. Meet each student individually and discuss why they are not attending
E. Notify the medical school

Question 199:

You are on the orthopaedic team. You frequently notice that the consultants use sexist and expletive language during the morning meeting when discussing patients. The registrars also join in. You and your fellow FY1 find the language uncomfortable.

Rank the actions below in order of most appropriate to least appropriate:

A. Speak to a consultant on your previous rotation about how to proceed
B. Send an email discreetly to your consultant raising the issue
C. Do nothing as they will be writing your review at the end of the rotation
D. Send an email to the matron of orthopaedics raising the issue
E. Participate in the behaviour to gain favour of the consultants

Question 200:

You are the colorectal FY1 on a busy surgical firm. You are needed in theatre to assist with an appendicectomy. The last time you were in theatre you passed out and have been too scared to go back since.

Rank the actions below in order of most appropriate to least appropriate:

A. Go to theatre as you have been personally asked
B. Say you will go to theatre but then do not. Claim that you were too busy and forgot if questioned
C. Say you are too busy on the ward
D. Explain to the registrar why you do not want to go to theatre
E. Ask a colleague to go to theatre and take a handover of their jobs

Question 201:

You are the breast surgery FY1. You find that the workload is very light and you are using your time to complete projects and audits in the doctor's mess. However, the FY1s on the other surgical teams have put in an official complaint to the foundation programme director about you, stating that you spend all your time in the mess and do not help them out. They have never asked you for help in person. The foundation programme director has called to see you.

Rank the actions below in order of most appropriate to least appropriate:

A. Explain to the foundation programme director that you are using your time productively
B. Send an email to all the other surgical FY1s telling them what you are actually doing in the doctor's mess
C. Ignore their complaint, assuming it was borne from jealousy
D. Offer to help the other FY1sE. Continue to spend all of your time doing your projects but on the ward

Question 202:
You have been volunteered by your peers to become the next doctors mess president. However, a colleague of yours also wants the position. The medical education team co-elects both of you. However, you have not liked your colleague since an incident at medical school. The feeling is mutual.

Rank the actions below in order of most appropriate to least appropriate:

A. Try to renew the friendship during the position
B. Resign from your post as mess president
C. Discuss the problem with your co-president
D. Discuss the problem with the medical education team
E. Send a message to the doctors asking them to vote for one or other of you

Question 203:
You are working a Saturday shift as the surgical FY2. No registrar or SHO turns up for work at 9AM. You are sent to A & E by the consultant to start seeing new patients. Nobody has arrived to assist you by 11AM.

Rank the actions below in order of most appropriate to least appropriate:

A. Continue as normal as you have been revising for the post graduate exams so feel you are competent enough
B. Make a meticulous list and ask the night registrar to review all of the patients
C. Notify the site practitioners or general manager
D. Call the consultant for advice to review your patients
E. Refuse to see any patients without a registrar

Question 204:
You are mentoring three medical students on your gastroenterology firm. You know one of them from medical school and are very good friends. One day they approach you on the ward and divulge that they have romantic feelings for you.

Rank the actions below in order of most appropriate to least appropriate:

A. Begin to pursue a relationship with them
B. Refuse to acknowledge their feelings, pretend that nothing has been said and continue as normal
C. Explain that as their mentor it would be inappropriate to take this further
D. Contact the medical education team to notify them of the situation
E. Ask the medical education team to change them off of your firm

Question 205:

You return to work after a weekend and are notified that one of your chronically unwell patients has passed away over the weekend. The patient was stable on Friday when you finished work. You are asked to fill in the death certificate and cremation paperwork.

Rank the actions below in order of most appropriate to least appropriate:

A. Email the on-call team present at the weekend to find out what happened
B. Fill in the death certificate
C. Call the patient's family to give your condolences and find out what happened
D. Read through the notes from over the weekend
E. Discuss with your consultant about what to write

Question 206:

The hospital is on high-alert after several patients recently acquired MRSA. The infection control team is regularly checking hand hygiene and ensuring that staff are "bare below the elbows". You remember that your registrar always wears a wrist-watch when examining patients.

Rank the actions below in order of most appropriate to least appropriate:

A. Notify your consultant
B. Notify the nurse in charge
C. Notify infection control
D. Monitor the situation over the next few days
E. Tell your registrar to remove their watch as they are breaching the infection control policy

Question 207:

Your registrar asks you to book a CT scan for a patient that they saw earlier. It is an extremely busy day and you haven't seen the patient yourself. You book the scan but are then called by the consultant radiologist asking for more details.

Rank the actions below in order of most appropriate to least appropriate:

A. Go and find the notes, read up on the patient, then call the radiologist back
B. Call your registrar and ask them for further details, then call the radiologist back
C. Discuss the patient's symptoms and invent some physical examination findings
D. Explain that you had not seen the patient and therefore would be unable to answer his questions
E. Ask your registrar to call the radiologist back

Question 208:

You review a patient who has had an elective hip replacement with your registrar on the morning ward round and deem her "medically fit for discharge". Due to hospital pressures, the nursing staff are keen to discharge her so they can get the bed ready for another patient. However, the patient calls you back and says they are not ready to go home as they live alone and do not have any support.

Rank the actions below in order of most appropriate to least appropriate:

A. Ask the nursing staff to arrange a 'package of care' for the patient
B. Speak to the bed manager to say that it is unlikely that the patient is going home
C. Explain that she is medically fit and can go home
D. Say that if she stays she will get a hospital acquired infection
E. Ask the patient about their concerns

Question 209:

One of your patients with end-stage heart failure is coming to the end of their life. The team is struggling with symptom control despite palliative care input. The patient states that he would like to go to a hospice to die. However, the family would like them to stay in hospital.

Rank the actions below in order of most appropriate to least appropriate:

A. See how events unfold over the next few days
B. Explore the patient's reasons for wanting to go to a hospice
C. Explore the family's reasons for wanting the patient to stay in hospital
D. Arrange a best-interests meeting with the multidisciplinary team
E. Ask the palliative care team to discuss hospice care with the patient

Question 210:

A patient is admitted with back pain. Their scan reports are strongly suspicious of cancer in the bones but the primary site is still unknown. The patient calls you over and asks you to explain the scan results and give the diagnosis.

Rank the actions below in order of most appropriate to least appropriate:

A. Explain that they will be fine as nothing of note was found
B. Explain that you will chase the results and ask a senior to discuss them
C. Explain that the scans have been done but you are still awaiting the report
D. Explore their ideas, concerns and expectations
E. Explain that they may need further investigations before a diagnosis can be made

Question 211:

A patient who was admitted overnight on the medical take has had their regular medications prescribed. However, the nurse notifies you on the ward round that they have been unable to obtain one of the cardiovascular medications as it is not in the hospital formulary.

Rank the actions below in order of most appropriate to least appropriate:

A. Search the BNF for an alternate drug for that condition and prescribe that
B. Ask the patient's family to bring in their medications from home and use those
C. Ask the pharmacist what to prescribe instead
D. Cross off the medication completely
E. Omit the medication until discharge

Question 212:

You are an FY1 on the acute assessment ward. A religious festival is coming up. You are working alone on the ward but would like to take the day off as annual leave. You approach your consultant and broach the subject but they dismiss it as you are the only one covering the job.

Rank the actions below in order of most appropriate to least appropriate:

A. Discuss the issue with your designated clinical supervisor
B. Notify your educational supervisor
C. Accept that you cannot take annual leave
D. Take the day off as sick leave
E. Seek legal advice from your defence union regarding religious discrimination

Question 213:

You are a new FY1 on your shadowing week. You are following an FY1 on the neurosurgical firm. After the ward round, they give you the bleep and leave. They state that you should do the job like they've also had to do it "without support", and that it would be "character building".

Rank the actions below in order of most appropriate to least appropriate:

A. Refuse to do the jobs and leave with the FY1 you are shadowing as your role is to follow them everywhere they go and do what they do
B. Notify the medical education department that your FY1 has left
C. Ask the nursing staff for help
D. Get on with the jobs as there is no one else to do them
E. Notify the neurosurgical SHO that you need help with the jobs

Question 214:

You are the anaesthetics FY1. You are being supervised in the insertion of a central line by one of the consultant anaesthetists. The consultant has asked you to go and consent the patient.

Rank the actions below in order of most appropriate to least appropriate:

A. Go and consent the patient as you are performing the procedure
B. Ask the anaesthetic SHO to consent the patient
C. Ask the anaesthetic consultant to consent the patient
D. Do not fill out a consent form as it is not required for this procedure
E. Explain that you are unable to consent the patient

Question 215:

You are on the acute medical unit. You have prescribed an amiodarone infusion to medically cardiovert a patient. However, whilst driving home you realise that you have prescribed the wrong dose due to a miscalculation.

Rank the actions below in order of most appropriate to least appropriate:

A. Cross out the dose in the morning
B. Call the ward and inform the nursing staff not to give the infusion
C. Notify the on-call registrar
D. Fill in an incident report
E. Call the on-call FY1 and ask them to review and amend the prescription as appropriate

Question 216:

You are asked by your registrar to perform a lumbar puncture on a severely confused patient because the registrar is busy at a cardiac arrest. You have performed the procedure many times and there are no contraindications to performing it. However, you are concerned about performing it on someone who lacks capacity.

Rank the actions below in order of most appropriate to least appropriate:

A. Refuse to perform the procedure
B. Contact the next of kin to discuss the procedure
C. Call the consultant and ask them to perform it
D. Perform the lumbar puncture as it is in the patient's best interests
E. Ask the medical registrar to perform the procedure

Question 217:

You are an FY2 and called to see a patient who has been admitted from A & E with a paracetamol overdose. They have been medically treated but keep stating they want to leave so they can "jump off of a bridge."

Rank the actions below in order of most appropriate to least appropriate:

A. Ask security to restrain the patient
B. Talk to the patient directly and ask them to stay
C. Allow the patient to leave as they have capacity
D. Section the patient under the mental health act
E. Call the patients next of kin and ask them to talk to the patient

Question 218:

You are the orthopaedic SHO on call and seeing a two-year-old in paediatric A & E. They have a fracture of their little finger- your registrar feels that this is a very strange injury for a child due to the force required to sustain it. Your concerns are mirrored by the paediatric team.

Rank the actions below in order of most appropriate to least appropriate:

A. Notify the doctor responsible for child protection
B. Perform a full examination of the child
C. Notify the police
D. Treat the patient and then discharge them
E. Question the parents regarding the mechanism of injury

Question 219:

You are the FY1 covering all surgical wards on a night shift. Your registrar and SHO are both on site but work 24 hours on call. They are tired after a busy day and are sleeping in the on call room. You are called to the ward as the nursing staff cannot cannulate a patient who has had back surgery. They need intravenous antibiotics for postoperative meningitis. You fail to cannulate twice.

Rank the actions below in order of most appropriate to least appropriate:

A. Call the anaesthetist to cannulate the patient
B. Omit the antibiotics until the morning
C. Attempt cannulation a third time
D. Wake your SHO and ask them to attempt cannulation
E. Wake your registrar and ask them to attempt cannulation

Question 220:

A heterosexual patient attends your genitourinary medicine clinic for the results of their HIV test. They are married but engaged in an extramarital sexual encounter whilst away on holiday. They are HIV positive. After counselling, they tell you that they don't want their partner to know.

Rank the actions below in order of most appropriate to least appropriate:

A. Notify the patient's partner
B. Explain to the patient that their partner is at risk if they are not informed
C. Convince them to use barrier protection if they are not going to tell their partner
D. Do not offer them treatment unless they tell their partner
E. Explain that you have a duty to tell their partner regardless of their consent

Question 221:

You have a forty-year-old patient in the intensive care unit who had a severe head injury. The patient is on the organ donor register and was declared brain dead this morning. The family do not want his organs donated.

Rank the actions below in order of most appropriate to least appropriate:

A. Dismiss the family's wishes
B. Notify the transplant team as this was the patient's wish
C. Notify the transplant team as it is in the public interest that these organs are used
D. Contact the specialist nurse for organ donation
E. Respect the family's wishes

Question 222:

You are the FY1 on orthogeriatrics. You feel that you have not had the senior SHO support that you have needed. Your SHO is always in the hospital coffee shop or library, stating that they are revising for upcoming membership exams. You have to pick up any extra work.

Choose the **THREE** most appropriate options.

A. Continue to pick up the extra work so that patient safety is not compromised
B. Directly discuss your concerns with the colleague involved
C. Ask other team members if they have similar concerns
D. Inform your registrar of your concerns
E. Report your SHO to the GMC
F. Explain to your SHO that they should not be revising during work hours when there are jobs to do
G. Document your concerns but take no further action at the present time
H. Ignore it as they are rotating jobs soon

Question 223:

You are the only FY1 on the Intensive Care Unit on your first rotation. You feel you are not getting any value from the rotation as you are only given the menial administrative tasks. You aren't being involved in clinical decision making or gaining experience in clinical skills.

Choose the **THREE** most appropriate options.

A. Speak to your supervising consultant
B. Ask the more senior trainees to help you with the more menial jobs
C. Organise teaching for the trainees from the consultants on Intensive Care related topics
D. Do nothing as the job is only 4 months long
E. Speak to your educational supervisor
F. Speak to the foundation programme director
G. Help to write some structured learning aims and objectives with a logbook for the rotation and discuss them with your clinical supervisor

Question 224:

You are on the acute medical take with a very senior SHO. They are covering for a registrar who is sick. The shift is very busy and they have admitted a patient with a lower respiratory tract infection. You are called by the nursing staff on the wards saying that they have prescribed a penicillin based antibiotic but the patient is stating that they are allergic to it.

Choose the **THREE** most appropriate options.

A. Go and review the patient clinically
B. Ask the patient about their allergy history
C. Give the drug as the drug chart does not state any allergies
D. Inform the consultant on call about the error
E. Complete an incident report
F. Do nothing as you have not seen the patient and it is not your responsibility
G. Advise the nursing staff not to give the antibiotic
H. Amend the prescription to a safer, alternative antibiotic

Question 225:

You are one of the surgical house officers. You are monitoring one of your patients for refeeding syndrome. On the ward round you tell the consultant that the electrolyte levels are normal, as stated on your handover sheet. However, later the nursing staff ask you to review the electrolyte results again as the lab has called saying they are abnormal. You notice that the potassium is very low.

Choose the **THREE** most appropriate options.

A. Change the details on your handover sheet
B. Inform your team of the correct results
C. Notify your consultant of the error
D. Inform the patient of the mistake
E. Instigate appropriate treatment
F. Repeat the electrolytes as they may be erroneous
G. Clinically review the patient
H. Ask a colleague to review the patient so that you can save face

Question 226:

You are about to finish your shift and handover. You are bleeped by a nurse who asks you to finish a discharge summary as the pharmacy closes at 5PM. You know that the patient is complex and the summary will take at least 20 minutes resulting in you finishing late.

Rank the actions below in order of most appropriate to least appropriate:

A. Ignore the request as you can do it tomorrow
B. Handover the discharge summary as you know pharmacy will have closed before it is finished anyway
C. Go to the ward and complete the discharge summary then go to handover
D. Ask the FY1 that you would handover to, to meet you on your ward whilst you do the discharge summary
E. Notify your registrar of the jobs that need to be handed over and then finish the discharge summary

Question 227:

You are one of the oncology juniors and have a patient with neutropaenic sepsis. You prescribed a medication for them last night to boost their immune system but when you arrive in the morning it has not been given. You clearly remember handing it over to the nursing team.

Rank the actions below in order of most appropriate to least appropriate:

A. Send an email to the nurse in charge last night asking why it wasn't given
B. Notify the senior sister immediately
C. Submit an incident report
D. Watch the nursing staff dispense and give the medication
E. Notify your consultant that the medication was not given

Question 228:

You are called by the biochemistry lab to say that the blood you collected for an elective pre-operative admission has spilled into the bag as the lid wasn't applied correctly. They need a new blood sample. It is near the end of the shift and you are busy in A & E seeing an unwell patient with your SHO.

Rank the actions below in order of most appropriate to least appropriate:

A. Ask the nursing staff to kindly take the blood
B. Leave the current patient as your SHO is there to go and retake the blood
C. Handover to the night team to take the bloods
D. Put bloods out for the morning phlebotomy round
E. Ask your registrar to take the bloods

Question 229:

You are on a very rapid surgical ward round seeing all the newly admitted patients. One patient with an intra-abdominal infection needs antibiotics but is penicillin-allergic. You do not know the second line agent to prescribe and your consultant has moved on to the next patient.

Choose the **THREE** most appropriate options.

A. Prescribe a penicillin antibiotic anyway as it's likely a very minor allergy.
B. Come back to the patient later to prescribe the correct antibiotic using the BNF
C. Ask your SHO if they know the appropriate drug
D. Prescribe a drug but don't sign it. Tell the nurses that you will come back and check it later in the BNF
E. Ask the ward pharmacist what their recommendation is
F. Do not prescribe the antibiotic as you can do it tomorrow when the ward round is done by the registrar
G. Search the hospital formulary quickly to find the protocol and prescribe it
H. Ask a fellow FY1 what they would prescribe and prescribe that

Question 230:

A patient has received bad news about a suspected cancer diagnosis and the plan from thereon. However, they have not understood. They keep asking, "Is it lung cancer?" The nursing staff call you to re-explain what was said to the patient. You were not there when the patient received the news.

Choose the **THREE** most appropriate options.

A. Recommend the patient asks the senior doctors tomorrow on the ward round
B. Ask a senior to speak to the patient and re-discuss the news
C. Ask the nursing staff to contact a senior to re-discuss the news
D. Establish a baseline to see what they currently understand
E. Print off a patient information leaflet about lung cancer and give that to the patient
F. Explain the news to the next of kin and then ask them to explain it to the patient
G. Speak to the patient and explain that they have cancer but not of the lung
H. Say to the patient you haven't got the experience to answer their questions but will find someone who does

Question 231:

A patient is admitted with urosepsis. They are deteriorating despite aggressive treatment and are becoming less responsive. The patient isn't for escalation beyond ward based care but the family are unaware of this. One evening, the patient stops responding and a cardiac arrest call is made. You and other members of the crash team arrive at the patient's bedside and the son is there. He does not wish to leave the room during the resuscitation attempt.

Choose the **THREE** most appropriate options.

A. Ask him again if he wishes to stay once CPR has commenced
B. Ask him to stand in the corner and not disrupt anyone
C. Explain to him that resuscitation is unlikely to be successful
D. Designate a member of the ward staff to stay with him
E. Use him to get more information about the family's burial wishes
F. Escort him out yourself saying he is in the way
G. Do nothing as he isn't bothering you
H. Ask the nurse in charge to escort him out of the room

Question 232:

You are asked to see a complex medical patient in general surgery clinic. However, there are neither medical notes nor a referral letter. They have been waiting three months for this appointment. When you explain this, the patient and her partner become extremely angry.

Choose the **THREE** most appropriate options.

A. List the patient for surgery. State that you will review them with their notes when they are admitted
B. Proceed to take a history to ascertain why they have come
C. Make another appointment for them to attend
D. Fill out an incident report
E. Call the GP surgery and ask them to fax over another copy of the referral letter and a medical summary
F. Refuse to continue the consultation without the notes
G. Apologise to the patient for the administrative error
H. Ask the patient to submit a formal complaint

Question 233:

You are an FY1 attending a simulation course with three other FY1s and four newly qualified nurses. It is the first time that the nurses are doing simulation. All the doctors have substantial simulation experience from their medical school. After one challenging scenario with an aggressive patient, the nursing student with you breaks down in tears.

Choose the **THREE** most appropriate options.

A. Speak to the nurse after the session to debrief about it
B. Ask the other nurses to go and speak to her
C. Ask your colleagues what to do
D. Ask another FY1 talk to her
E. Notify the facilitators of the session
F. Fill in an incident form as the nurse may not be fit to practice
G. Give her some space and time to cry
H. Give her a hug

Question 234:

A patient is admitted Friday night with a severe chest infection and delirium. You do not know their regular medications but are aware that they have a complex cardiac background.

Choose the **THREE** most appropriate options.

A. Prescribe the relevant medications pertinent to their past medical history
B. Look at the hospital guidelines for the conditions they have and prescribe the first line agents
C. Contact the next of kin and try to obtain a drug history
D. Check the ambulance sheet for any medications
E. Check their previous discharge summaries for any medications
F. Ask the pharmacist on call to search their GP medication records the next day
G. Do not prescribe anything
H. Prescribe drugs to treat the infection but nothing else. Ask the team taking over on Monday morning to ask the GP for the patient's medications.

Question 235:

You are the FY2 on Hepatobilliary surgery and assisting in a liver resection for a patient with Hepatitis C. You obtain a blood-splash injury to the eyes when there is accidental damage to a blood vessel.

Choose the **THREE** most appropriate options.

A. Submit an incident report
B. Go to accident and emergency immediately
C. Take the patient's blood intra-operatively and send them for virology screen
D. De-scrub and use the emergency eye wash
E. Notify occupational health
F. Continue with the operation as you are needed
G. Ask the nursing staff to take your blood and send it for testing
H. Ask someone to take the patient's blood after they have recovered from the anaesthetic and have given consent

Question 236:

You are on call on the Friday before the bank holiday weekend. You want to leave two hours early to drive home to see your parents, which is five hours away.

Choose the **THREE** most appropriate options.

A. Call in sick and leave for those two hours
B. Ask another FY1 who is on call the next day to cover the last two hours as their weekend is ruined anyway
C. Swap the entire shift with someone so you can get away on time
D. Complete the whole shift and drive home the next day
E. Abandon your plans to go home for the weekend
F. Ask your SHO to cover you for the last two hours and leave
G. Give a telephone handover to the night FY1 and tell them where you are leaving the bleep and go
H. Ask the night FY1 to come in two hours early to cover you and say you will do one of their other on calls in return

Question 237:

You are working in a small district general hospital. One of your SHOs is a trust grade from abroad who speaks limited English. You are finding that communication is becoming a barrier to effective teamwork and handover.

Choose the **THREE** most appropriate options.

A. Do nothing as your rotation will be ending shortly
B. Speak to the SHO directly to address your concerns
C. Speak to your educational supervisor
D. Notify your service manager about the ongoing problems
E. Speak to your supervising consultant
F. Speak to the medical education team to arrange communication sessions for the SHO
G. Notify your registrar
H. Report the SHO to the GMC

Question 238:

You are an FY2 working in accident and emergency. A patient who speaks very little English comes in after being assaulted. The police suspect it to be a racially motivated attack. The patient confides in you that he is an illegal immigrant as his student visa has recently expired and he has not been granted another one. He says he cannot afford to pay for any care.

Choose the **THREE** most appropriate options.

A. Ask your consultant to review the patient
B. Treat the patient regardless of his ability to pay
C. Ask the nurse in charge what to do
D. Refuse to treat the patient until they can provide insurance documents
E. Notify the police the patient is an illegal immigrant
F. Treat the patient and then notify your consultant that the patient will not be able to pay for their care
G. Ask the hospital team in charge of private healthcare to come and see the patient to discuss their treatment
H. Ask a colleague to see the patient

Question 239:

You are in urology clinic with a consultant who is watching you perform a consultation. You see a foreign couple- the gentleman has been referred for consideration of an elective vasectomy. He does not speak any English and his wife is the translator. You explain the risks of the procedure including that it is unlikely to be reversible. From his body language you can tell he is a bit apprehensive but his wife says that he wants to do it and asks for the consent form. You are concerned she is not directly translating what he is saying.

Choose the **THREE** most appropriate options.

A. Try and find a staff member to translate for you
B. Reiterate to the wife she needs to translate word for word otherwise the consent will not be valid
C. Fill in a consent form and ask him to sign it
D. Arrange a formal translator for a future clinic and invite them back to it
E. Ask the consultant to step outside with you and ask for their advice on how to proceed
F. List him for the procedure but do not consent him for it
G. Use an online translator to communicate with the patient after asking the wife to step outside whilst you "examine the patient"
H. Discharge him from clinic- stating that he did not want the procedure based on his body language

Question 240:

You have just become an FY1 doctor and are on the general surgery team. You are asked to see a young gentleman who is suspected to have appendicitis. You recognise the name as someone you went to university with.

Choose the **THREE** most appropriate options.

A. Send a message to your friends saying that he is in hospital and they should come and see him
B. Explain to the registrar that you know this patient
C. Take a history but do not examine him to save him embarrassment
D. Go and see the patient regardless but don't mention that you may know them
E. Ask the patient if they mind that you are the doctor looking after them
F. Ask the SHO to see the patient instead
G. Order some appropriate investigations from afar but do not review him
H. Pop your head in and see if you recognise the patient. Walk away if you do

Question 241:

You are the on-call cardiology FY2 and asked to see a patient who has chest pain after their angiogram. You aren't the patient's normal doctor. The night team told you that the patient has a background of significant cardiovascular co-morbidities. The patient is sat up in bed talking when you arrive.

Choose the **THREE** most appropriate options in order of action.

A. Document your findings clearly, including a plan of action
B. Ask the nursing staff to perform observations
C. Take a full history from the patient about the chest pain
D. Assess the patient from an ABCDE approach
E. Look through the notes to get a background about the patient before seeing them
F. Order appropriate investigations
G. Call the medical registrar for advice
H. Call the patient's family

Question 242:

You have two male patients on the ward with the same surname in the same bay. One of them needs a Computed Tomography scan of their chest which you arranged yesterday. Unfortunately, you arranged it for the wrong patient and you only discover this once the wrong patient returns from radiology.

Choose the **THREE** most appropriate options.

A. Notify the nurse in charge of the mistake
B. Apologise to the patient who didn't have the scan
C. Submit an incident report
D. Order a CT scan for the other patient
E. Apologise to the patient who had the scan
F. Notify your consultant of the mistake
G. Notify radiology the wrong patient has had a scan
H. Do not tell anyone as it's not a big problem. Ensure you reorder the scan for the correct patient.

Question 243:

You have a particularly difficult first month as an FY1 with a high burden of on-calls. Over the past few days you have started to feel unwell. During the morning ward round, you feel feverish and nauseous and have to excuse yourself to vomit in the toilet.

Choose the **THREE** most appropriate options.

A. Ask the nursing staff for anti-sickness medications and continue
B. Ask your SHO to prescribe anti-sickness medications for you to pick up from pharmacy
C. Notify human resources of the issue
D. Notify your consultant that you are not feeling well
E. Continue as normal as leaving is a sign of weakness
F. Leave work directly from the toilet without telling anyone as you risk infecting patients if you go back on the ward round
G. Restrict yourself to paperwork for the day and do not go into patients' rooms
H. Go to accident and emergency for some anti-sickness medication and then continue with the day

Question 244:

You, Jenny and Tom are FY1s on the respiratory team. Jenny says that she has noticed that Tom has been falling asleep on the job. She is concerned that he is not sleeping well and that this is affecting his clinical performance, putting pressure on yourselves. You have not witnessed this before.

Choose the **THREE** most appropriate options.

A. Explain that you have not seen Tom acting this way before
B. Ask Jenny to speak directly to the Tom
C. Speak directly to the Tom; ask if he is feeling unusually tired at work
D. Inform a senior colleague about what has been happening yourself
E. Advise Jenny to speak to a senior colleague about her concerns
F. Ask other FY1s to see if they have noticed anything
G. Ask Jenny to ask the junior doctors to see if they have noticed anything
H. Tell Jenny to email the consultant with her concerns

Question 245:
You are an FY1 working on the Acute Medical Unit. There is an intoxicated patient who has suffered a head injury after a night out. He was admitted as the team were unable to fully assess his neurological status due to his inebriation. He is becoming increasingly aggressive and threatening both staff and patients.

Choose the **THREE** most appropriate options.

A. Call security
B. Try and calm the patient yourself
C. Apologise to other patients in the bay and ensure that none have come to harm
D. Ask the nursing staff to hold him down whilst you sedate him
E. Move other patients out of the bay
F. Say to the patient that you will discharge him if he does not calm down
G. Tell the patient that his behaviour is inappropriate and will not be tolerated
H. Ask the nursing staff to calm the patient down

Question 246:
You receive a call from a consultant microbiologist. They state that one of your patients has grown MRSA on a wound swab and ask you to start the appropriate treatment, which you do. However, on the morning ward round the ward consultant disagrees with this management and tells you to change the antibiotics.

Choose the **THREE** most appropriate options.

A. Ask the pharmacist for their opinion
B. Ask the consultant's reasoning for wanting to change the antibiotics
C. Ask your consultant to call microbiology
D. Change the antibiotics as directed
E. Explain to your consultant why microbiology wants the current regimen
F. Say you will change the antibiotics but then don't
G. Call microbiology and notify them of your consultant's wishes
H. Ask the patient which antibiotics they want

Question 251:

You are the FY1 on geriatrics. It is Saturday morning and you have the weekend off. You suddenly realise that you forgot to request an INR for a patient you are loading on warfarin. The on-call doctor will need an up to date INR to appropriately prescribe the correct warfarin dose.

Rank the actions below in order of most appropriate to least appropriate:

A. Go to the hospital and bleed the patient for an INR. Wait the two hours a non-urgent sample takes in the lab, prescribe the Warfarin based on the INR and then leave
B. Go to the hospital and bleed the patient for an INR, inform the lab that this is an urgent sample, prescribe the Warfarin based on the INR and then leave
C. Call your ward and ask them to bleep the on-call doctor and explain the situation. The on-call doctor can then bleed the patient early in the day to obtain the INR value needed to prescribe the Warfarin in time for the 7PM drug round
D. Call your friend who is currently on-call for surgery to go and bleed the patient as a favour to you, so no one discovers your mistake.
E. Do nothing; when the on-call doctor goes to prescribe the warfarin they will find there is no up to date INR and they will bleed the patient then.

Question 252:

You are obliged to attend 70% of your weekly one-hour teaching sessions to pass FY1. Your friend is rarely able to leave the ward to attend teaching because of his heavy work load and unsupportive seniors. He asks you to sign his name on the register when you attend teaching to bolster his attendance record.

Rank the actions below in order of most appropriate to least appropriate:

A. Sign his name in the register as it's unfortunate that he is too busy to attend and would be unfair for him to fail the year. Your next rotation is a notoriously busy one so hopefully he will return the favour
B. Advise him that you signing the register is dishonest. He would be better to raise the issue of his unsupportive seniors and busy job to the head of the foundation programme so changes can be made for him and further trainees.
C. Tell him you have signed him in but then don't
D. Contact the head of the foundation programme as his advocate and explain his predicament
E. Offer to go with him to discuss it with the head of the foundation programme but agree to sign the register this time

Question 253:

You have to be witnessed performing twenty procedural skills to be signed off FY1 as competent. Your SHO tells you to send him the forms that need signing for the basic procedures. He isn't going to watch you do them as he knows you do them daily.

Rank the actions below in order of most appropriate to least appropriate:

A. Thank him and send a form for just one procedure that you think will be the hardest to get signed off
B. Thank him and send the forms for procedural skills you are confident and comfortable with
C. Thank him but explain this is dishonest and could get both of you in trouble
D. Report him to the deanery as this is a probity issue
E. Thank him but explain that you would feel more comfortable if he observed you performing the procedures first. If he refuses, seek alternative colleagues to observe you

Question 254:

You are the FY1 on Geriatrics. Your consultant informed you yesterday that she is in meetings until the afternoon so expects you to get on with your own ward round until she arrives at 1400. You are stuck in traffic on the motorway and know you are going to be at least twenty minutes late to work. You are the only doctor on your ward today.

Rank the actions below in order of most appropriate to least appropriate:

A. You can make up the lost time by not having lunch so you will still finish your ward by 1400.
B. Call the ward and inform them that you are on your way but stuck in traffic. Give them your mobile number and assure them that if any problems crop up before you arrive then they should call you.
C. Call the ward and inform them that you are on your way but stuck in traffic. Give them the bleep number of the doctor on the adjacent geriatric ward and assure them that if any problems crop up before you arrive then they should contact them.
D. Contact your consultant via switch board to alert her that you will be twenty minutes late
E. Call the ward and inform them that you are on your way but stuck in traffic. Instruct them to contact the consultant via switch board if there are any problems with the patients before you arrive

Question 255:

You are the general surgery FY1. You want to be a psychiatrist whilst your fellow FY1 who you work with on the ward wants to be a surgeon. They take every opportunity to assist in theatre, often leaving you to do all the ward jobs. You often leave late as a result.

Rank the actions below in order of most appropriate to least appropriate:

A. Discuss with the operating surgeon that it is unfair for your colleague to leave you to do all the ward work
B. Discuss with your fellow FY1 that you don't mind him going to theatre but he must only go once his half of the jobs are done
C. Just get on with it as you find theatre boring anyway
D. Discuss the situation with your FY1 colleague; alternate who goes to theatre and who stays on the ward. Even though ultimately you don't want to be a surgeon, it is good for your learning to assist in theatre especially as they will be operating on patients you will look after post-operatively
E. Contact your medical defence union as this is bullying in the workplace

Question 256:

You are the FY1 on Urology. You have never inserted a catheter nor seen one done and are nervous about it. Your colleague working on the same ward confides that she finds venepuncture and cannulation challenging. She suggests that when dividing up jobs, you should always do venepuncture/cannulation and she should always do the catheters.

Rank the actions below in order of most appropriate to least appropriate:

A. This is fair distribution of work because on a urology ward there are equal amounts of both venepuncture/cannulas and catheters to do. Working to the individuals' strengths is a pillar of good team work
B. Decline her offer and just give it a go - you are bound to work it out after repeated attempts
C. Put time aside each day to practise the skills you are weak at; ask her to demonstrate catheterisation and then assist you doing one and vice versa
D. Decline her offer as this is not appropriate as qualified doctors. Each time you are asked to catheterise have one attempt and if you fail ask your colleague to complete the procedure
E. Book in a session in the clinical skills lab for the pair of you where you can both safely practice

Question 257:

It is 8PM and you have just finished your on-call shift on the Medical Assessment Unit. You have plans to meet your boyfriend's parents for dinner for the first time. Your colleague, who should have arrived to take over from you, is already late. They have been approximately thirty minutes late to handover every day this week.

Rank the actions below in order of most appropriate to least appropriate:

A. Write out a list of jobs to handover, tape them to the computer screen in the office where you meet, leave the bleep by the keyboard, and then leave for the day
B. Call her and enquire about her whereabouts. Ascertain how long she will be and then ring your boyfriend to let him know that you will be late to dinner. On her arrival speak to her about her reasons for being late and how it affects others around her. Hand over fully, then leave
C. Call your boyfriend and let him know that you will be late for dinner. It has only been 30 minutes on other days and you have a duty of care to your patients. On her arrival, hand over fully then leave.
D. Leave her a message saying you have given the handover list of jobs and the bleep to the SHO to carry until she arrives, then leave for the day
E. Call your educational supervisor to discuss her behaviour. This has happened every night this week and perhaps she needs help

Question 258:

You are the FY1 on general surgery. You notice on the morning ward round that your consultant smells of alcohol and looks dishevelled. You have heard the nurses gossiping that he's going through a divorce; his wife is a paediatrician in the same hospital.

Rank the actions below in order of most appropriate to least appropriate:

A. Ignore it as it isn't your business
B. Take the consultant aside and offer him a mint so that patients don't smell alcohol on his breath
C. Discuss the case with your registrar
D. Call your educational supervisor immediately
E. Confront the consultant and demand that they go home right now

Question 259:

You are the stroke FY1. A medical student working on your ward often comes to work with bracelets, a watch and dangly earrings. She also never ties her long hair up. The infection control policy states doctors should be bare below the elbow in all clinical areas.

Rank the actions below in order of most appropriate to least appropriate:

A. Inform her of the policy. It is now up to her to abide by the rule or not
B. Inform her of the policy. If she continues to ignore the rule then flag it to the ward matron
C. Inform her of the policy. If she continues to ignore the rule then flag it to the infection control team
D. Ignore the issue. If it's a problem then the ward matron would have informed her by now
E. Start wearing whatever you fancy to work as the policy is clearly not policed

Question 260:

You recently looked after an elderly female on your ward. Her son comes to the ward and thanks you for the care that you provided. He then tries to give you £500 as thanks.

Choose the **THREE** most appropriate actions to take in this situation:

A. Accept the money and ask him not to tell anyone about it
B. Accept the money and tell the ward staff about his gratitude
C. Refuse to take his money
D. Suggest that he buys biscuits for all of the ward staff with the money
E. Suggest that he donate the money to the ward fund
F. Thank him for his gesture - saying it is very kind of him but refuse the money
G. Accept the money and tell your supervisor you have done so
H. Suggest he buys you some flowers instead with the money as you cannot accept money

Question 261:

You are an SHO working in A & E. A patient attends following a non-fatal stab wound. He does not want you to talk to the police about what has happened and claims that he does not know his attacker.

Choose the **THREE** most appropriate actions to take in this situation:

A. Advise the patient that you have a duty to inform the police about the incident as other members of the public may be at risk
B. Advise the patient that you will not pass on any information about the incident to the police but try to persuade him to do so himself.
C. After you have acted, make sure you let the supervising emergency department consultant know what steps you have taken
D. Discuss the case with the emergency department consultant before acting
E. Do not report the incident to the police as doing so would breach the patient's confidentiality
F. Do not tell the patient that you have spoken to the police as he may be dangerous and could react in such a way as to endanger your safety or the safety of other staff and patients
G. Report the incident to the police but do not pass on the patient's name or address without his consent
H. Report the incident to the police, including the patient's name and address

Question 262:

You are an SHO working at a general practice surgery. You receive a call from social services requesting information on a young boy (not your patient). He has been taken into care because of alleged child abuse and they would like more details about his dad (your patient).

Choose the **THREE** most appropriate actions to take in this situation:

A. Inform your patient about the social services request
B. Ignore their request for the time being as you have more important patient issues to deal with first
C. Write back to social services asking them to write to the Chief Executive of your healthcare trust
D. Seek your patient's consent to disclose confidential information
E. Write back to social services and refuse their request as this would be a breach of patient confidentiality
F. Inform social services that they will need to obtain a court order first to have access to his records
G. Co-operate with social services regardless of whether or not your patient has consented to the information being handed over
H. Wait until your patient has consented before disclosing the information requested

Question 263:

You are a FY1 on general surgery. Your consultant asks you alter notes to cover up for a mistake that has been made by the surgical team.

Choose the **THREE** most appropriate actions to take in this situation:

A. Make the change requested by the consultant as you are worried that they may give you a bad reference otherwise
B. Refuse to make the entry
C. Make a note of the conversation that you had with the consultant and contact your defence union
D. Report the matter to the Clinical Director at the earliest opportunity
E. Inform the patient of the mistake and also the consultant's request
F. Inform the GMC
G. Inform the police as there are potential legal implications
H. Complete a critical incident form

Question 264:

You are the urology FY1. Your registrar looks unwell; she asks you to prescribe her some antibiotics as she has a UTI but does not have time to see her GP.

Choose the **THREE** most appropriate actions to take in this situation:

A. Advise her to see her GP for antibiotics
B. Advise her to go to the Emergency Department for antibiotics
C. Prescribe her antibiotics on a private prescription
D. Prescribe her antibiotics on a hospital prescription
E. Refuse to prescribe her any antibiotics as it is not appropriate
F. Tell her to prescribe her own antibiotics on a private prescription
G. Suggest that she takes some suitable antibiotics from the drug cupboard
H. Complete a chest x-ray form for her and suggest she sees if she has a chest infection before initiating any treatment

Question 265:

You have finished work two hours early and have no additional tasks to complete. All the notes are up to date and your patients appear stable. Your bleep works at home.

Choose the **THREE** most appropriate actions to take in this situation:

A. Stay on the ward
B. Go home
C. Go to the doctor's mess
D. Keep your bleep
E. Hand over your bleep to the ST1
F. Relax
G. Work on your audit
H. Offer to help your colleagues

Question 266:

You are on call for Paediatrics. You have seen a child who has presented to A & E several times in the past with unrelated problems. Today the child has a suspicious burn and bruises to his arm. You ask the father whether anyone could have hurt the child. The father gets angry and threatens to sue you.

Choose the **THREE** most appropriate actions to take in this situation:

A. Inform the consultant of the incident and ask for advice
B. Give reassurance to the father and treat the patient's injury appropriately
C. Let the father discharge the child from the hospital
D. Call the police and report the incident
E. Privately ask the mother whether there has been any abuse
F. Speak to the hospital legal team regarding the possibility of a lawsuit
G. Admit the child to the ward for further assessment
H. Report the family to social services

Question 267:

You are the general medicine FY1. You are exhausted as you've finished your night shift. You are preparing to go home when you receive a call from the day FY1. They are suffering from diarrhoea and vomiting and won't be coming into work. You are due to work the following night as well.

Choose the **THREE** most appropriate actions to take in this situation:

A. Tell the FY1 to pull himself together and come to work
B. Leave your bleep in a designated place
C. Let the site manager know that the day FY1 doctor is unable to come to the hospital
D. Head home as you are unsafe to continue working
E. Work as much of the day shift as you can before you cannot continue and then alert the responsible manager
F. Continue working to the best of your ability
G. Keep holding the bleep but decline to review patients as you are tired and unsafe
H. Ask the responsible manager to arrange cover so that you have sufficient time to sleep before returning to work

Question 268:

You are the orthopaedic FY1. A patient you saw last week in pre-assessment clinic arrived for surgery today. Whilst reviewing the notes, you realise that you had forgotten to listen to the heart. Today, you hear a murmur.

Choose the **THREE** most appropriate actions to take in this situation:

A. Ignore the murmur
B. Tell the anaesthetist that they may want to listen to the patient's heart
C. Document the murmur
D. Inform the patient of your findings and possible delay of surgery
E. Inform your consultant that the patient will need further investigations that are likely to delay the surgery
F. Contact the echo department to request an echo to be performed in the next fifteen minutes
G. Complete a critical incident form
H. Tell the consultant that the patient is ready for surgery

Question 269:

During a busy clinic, you overhear a ward clerk talking to one of the regular patients. She is making fun of a patient who came in earlier.

Choose the **THREE** most appropriate actions to take in this situation:

A. Firmly tell the ward clerk to stop the discussion there and then
B. Tell the ward clerk you will raise the issue with the clinic manager if it happens again
C. Raise the matter with the clinic manager
D. Apologise to other patients present and reassure them that it will not happen again
E. Draw the ward clerk away from the discussion by telling her that you need help with another patient then have a private word with her
F. Discuss the matter with your consultant
G. Document the issue in both patient's notes
H. Complete a critical incident form

Question 270:

You're an FY1 in paediatrics. A 16-year-old patient asks whether you could prescribe her the oral contraceptive pill (OCP) as she regularly has unprotected sex with her sixteen-year-old boyfriend. She asks that you do not tell her mother.

Choose the **THREE** most appropriate actions to take in this situation:

A. Prescribe the OCP
B. Ask the patient to see her local GP or the local sexual health/family planning clinic
C. Advise the patient that you can only prescribe or refer her to other services if she attends a local "safer sex" learning course
D. Inform her mother
E. Report the matter to social services
F. Do not prescribe the OCP
G. Tell the patient that you cannot prescribe the OCP whilst she is in hospital
H. Offer the patient some leaflets on safer sex

Question 271:

You are the cardiology FY1. Whilst rewriting a patient's drug chart, you notice that one of your colleagues has prescribed Furosemide **and** Bumetanide for a heart failure patient. The patient has had 6 doses of Furosemide but has not had any Bumetanide yet. You recently attended a teaching session where you learned that this is unsafe prescribing.

Choose the **THREE** most appropriate actions to take in this situation:

A. Call your colleague to explore why they've prescribed both drugs
B. Complete an incident form
C. Ignore it as they are unlikely to be approved by the ward pharmacist
D. Inform the patient and apologise on behalf of your colleague
E. Rewrite the drug chart without the Furosemide
F. Rewrite the drug chart without the Bumetanide
G. Review the medical notes and adjust the drug chart depending on the plan from your colleague
H. Review the patient and then discuss the incident with the ward registrar after

Question 272:

You are the orthopaedic SHO and working with a locum registrar. A patient presents with a fracture of the tibial shaft. You are convinced that the patient has compartment syndrome and requires urgent surgery. The registrar says that there is no evidence of compartment syndrome. He admits the patient for analgesia and observation. Four hours later, you find evidence of foot ischaemia. Again, the registrar says that there is no evidence of compartment syndrome.

Choose the **THREE** most appropriate actions to take in this situation:

A. Accept the registrar's opinion- he is more experienced and you have discharged your duty by asking them
B. After telling the registrar what you intend to do, phone the on-call orthopaedic consultant at home and raise your concerns with her
C. Ask the other on-call orthopaedic senior house officer, who is more experienced than you, to review the patient
D. Away from the bedside, attempt to explain the reasoning behind your diagnosis of compartment syndrome to the registrar and explore his justification for disagreeing with this
E. Document your disagreement with the registrar's opinion, the outcome of the discussion, and the steps you intend to take to solve the problem in the medical notes
F. Phone the on-call orthopaedic consultant at home and raise your concerns with her but do not tell the registrar that you plan to do this
G. Wait for the post-take ward round in the morning, when there will be an opportunity to gain a definitive opinion from the on-call consultant

Question 273:
You are an FY1 in paediatrics. You administer a tetanus vaccination to one of your patients and they are subsequently discharged. You later find that the vaccination had expired a year ago. The nurse who prepared the trolley blames you and threatens to fill an incident form against you.

Choose the **THREE** most appropriate actions to take in this situation:

A. Speak to the ward sister about the nurse's error and unprofessionalism
B. Explain to the parents what has happened but reassure them that it is unlikely that the error will cause any harm
C. Contact the parents at home to explain what has happened and advise that they should return if there are any concerns
D. Contact the parents at home and tell them that they need to return to casualty straight away, without causing undue alarm by only specifying that another injection is required
E. Speak to the nurse to discuss the incident and discourage her from completing an incident form
F. Respond to the nurse saying that you intend to do an incident form against her
G. Discuss the incident with the nurse and ward sister; ensure an incident form is completed
H. Seek advice from a consultant who happens to be on the ward but is not a member of your team

Question 274:
A nurse asks you to assess a patient who wants to self-discharge from the ward. The patient is likely to have lung cancer but hasn't had all their investigations yet. He is very agitated and borders on aggressive, which is making the nursing staff feel threatened.

Choose the **THREE** most appropriate actions to take in this situation:

A. Spend some time listening to the patient's concerns
B. Tell the patient that you are sorry that he is upset
C. Tell the patient that you understand how he feels
D. Explain to the patient that it is perfectly normal to be anxious about a possible diagnosis of lung cancer
E. Explain to the patient that it is important that he completes all the tests
F. Explain to the patient that if he leaves he could be putting himself at risk
G. Offer the patient help for his anxiety

Question 275:
A 90-year-old patient tells you that he is ready to die and no longer wants to take his statin.

Choose the **THREE** most appropriate actions to take in this situation:

A. Assess the patient's capacity
B. Ask him to explain why he feels he wants to die, offer support but explain to him that stopping this medication is unlikely to hasten his death
C. Offer to help him die
D. If he has capacity, explain that he is entitled to make his own decisions
E. Write a DNAR order for the patient
F. Inform his relatives
G. Give the patient details of a Swiss clinic that could help him die
H. Tell the patient that his decision is not rational and therefore you will act in his best interests and impose that he should continue treatment

Question 276:
You are the geriatrics FY1. An elderly patient with dementia is attempting to leave the ward. He has punched a nurse who tried to encourage him back to his bay. You do not believe that he has capacity.

Choose the **THREE** most appropriate actions to take in this situation:

A. Try to talk to the patient from a safe distance
B. Tackle the patient's legs and try to break his fall
C. Contact security urgently
D. Try to conduct an AMTS from a safe distance
E. Attend to the nurse's injuries as soon as it is appropriate to do so
F. Shout and wave at the patient to encourage him back into the ward
G. Sedate the patient with propofol for his own safety and the safety of others
H. Continue your work as agitated patients are a problem for the nursing team

Question 277:
You are the general surgery FY1. A patient is admitted with presumed liver disease, however, investigations show no evidence of liver disease. Your registrar tells the patient that the admitting team were "completely clueless".

Choose the **THREE** most appropriate actions to take in this situation:

A. Return to the patient after the ward round and apologise for the registrar's comment
B. Return to the patient after the ward round and clarify the registrar's comment. Explain that the admitting team did not have access to the investigation results
C. Ask a member of the admitting team about the discrepancies in the two management plans
D. Inform the patient that she can submit a written complaint about the registrar's comments
E. Confront the registrar after the ward round about the comment
F. Inform the consultant about the registrar's comment
G. Ask your SHO about advice on how to proceed
H. Ignore the comment and continue as normal

Question 278:

You are at lunch with a colleague who suddenly starts crying because she is not coping with her workload. She thinks that she is looking after too many patients, her consultant expects her to know too much, and the nurses are bullying her.

Choose the **THREE** most appropriate actions to take in this situation:

A. Advise her to take annual leave
B. Ask the nurses to be more supportive
C. Discuss her reasons for these feelings
D. Encourage her to seek professional counselling
E. Inform her educational supervisor that she is struggling
F. Offer to look after some of her patients
G. Offer to go with her to talk to her consultant
H. Suggest she discusses the issues with her FY2

Question 279:

You work with a registrar who is often unobtainable. Yet again you have bleeped him to review a very sick patient urgently and he has not turned up. Whenever you ask him where he's been his excuse is that his bleep must not be working.

Choose the **THREE** most appropriate actions to take in this situation:

A. Contact your consultant to inform him about the problem
B. Ignore the problem but make sure that whenever you require help you seek advice from an ST3 on another team
C. Ignore the problem but make sure that whenever you require help you seek advice from another FY1 doctor on your team
D. Initiate a meeting with the ST3 to get to the bottom of the problem
E. Ask some of the nurses whether they have heard the registrar's bleep going off so as to check if he's telling the truth
F. Complete a critical incident form
G. Complain to a senior nurse about the problem
H. Report the ST3 to the GMC

Question 280:

You are the orthopaedic FY1. A complex patient with multiple co-morbidities is admitted to your ward. They are in fast atrial fibrillation, cannot eat or drink, have 20kg weight loss and are short of breath at rest. They have not had any investigations or treatment.

Their observations are stable. Your registrar only seems concerned with their orthopaedic issues and ignores the other medical problems on the ward round. You are concerned that the patient is not receiving good medical care but realise that the orthopaedic team don't have the experience to manage the medical problems.

Rank the actions below in order of most appropriate to least appropriate:

A. Speak to the on call medical registrar and ask them for advice on the phone
B. Speak to the on call medical registrar and ask them to see the patient on the ward
C. Listen to your registrar as they are more experienced then you
D. Assess and treat the patient to the best of your ability
E. Speak to the on call orthopaedic registrar and ask them for advice on the phone

Question 281:

You are the on call respiratory FY1. During the shift you find your colleague taking a sip from a vodka bottle. Her shift does not finish for another three hours. She does not appear drunk.

Rank the actions below in order of most appropriate to least appropriate:

A. Offer to cover the remainder of her shift. Discuss the situation with your colleague and suggest she visits her GP or occupational health
B. Tell her that her behaviour in unacceptable as she is unsafe to treat patients and immediately report her to the ward registrar or consultant
C. Offer to cover the remainder of her shift and do nothing else
D. As your colleague does not appear drunk, let her continue working but tell her that you will talk to her educational supervisor if it happens again
E. As your colleague does not appear drunk, ignore the situation as it will embarrass her to discuss it with you

Question 282:

You are the respiratory FY1. One of the patients under your care died yesterday; your consultant states that you should put down pneumonia as the cause of death. You do not agree. Your consultant is now off site, and the patient's family are waiting for you to complete the death certificate.

Rank the actions below in order of most appropriate to least appropriate:

A. Discuss the case with the registrar
B. Speak to the coroner's office
C. Complete the death certificate with what you feel is a more appropriate entry
D. Refuse to complete the death certificate yourself
E. Adhere to the decision reached by your consultant

Question 283:

You have just started a job as an SHO in a new hospital. Your wife has a chest infection, and is not yet registered with a GP and has asked you to prescribe antibiotics.

Rank the actions below in order of most appropriate to least appropriate:

A. Prescribe the medication as a private prescription, and arrange for her to register with a GP the following week
B. Tell her to register with a GP locally
C. Prescribe the medication on a hospital take home prescription with her details on it
D. Prescribe the medication on a hospital take home prescription with one of your patient's details on it. Collect the medication from the hospital pharmacy
E. Ask one of your work colleagues to write a prescription on a hospital take home script without seeing your wife

Question 284:

Your best friend is on holiday abroad. During that period, her father is admitted in the hospital where you work, but in a different service. Your friend calls you and asks for information about her father as the hospital is refusing to give her any indication as to the nature of the illness or whether she needs to return from her holiday early.

Rank the actions below in order of most appropriate to least appropriate:

A. Ask your consultant for advice on what you should do
B. Tell your friend that you will raise the matter with her father's consultant
C. Ask your friend to give you written confirmation that you are permitted to request the information on her behalf
D. Tell your friend that you will ask her father to get in touch with her
E. Decline politely- tell your friend that her request would be in breach of regulations

Question 285:

Your consultant asks you whether you would be interested in doing an audit project. You are already doing an audit project for another consultant and you will not have enough time to do both.

Rank the actions below in order of most appropriate to least appropriate:

A. Refuse, explaining that you have another project to do but you ask your colleagues to see if any are interested
B. Refuse, saying that you are too busy with another audit project
C. Say that you might be interested but you need some more time to think about it; secretly hope they forget about asking you again
D. Agree to do the project and mentally plan to give up your free days to complete it
E. Agree you will do it as you don't wish to say no but plan to drag it out until you leave

Question 286:

You are the haematology FY1 on-call. You receive a call from the private wing of the hospital. You are asked to cannulate a patient for a blood transfusion. The ward nurse called the responsible consultant at home who told her to bleep you.

Rank the actions below in order of most appropriate to least appropriate:

A. Assess the urgency of the transfusion and prioritise according to your other tasks
B. Help if you are able but let the receptionist know that they should have somebody capable of cannulating patients on site
C. Contact a responsible person (e.g. the duty manager) to ask about the appropriateness of attending to tasks in the private wing
D. Cannulate the patient but leave an invoice with the receptionist for £80
E. Decline to re-site the cannula regardless of the clinical situation and suggest that the consultant comes in from home as it is their private patient

Question 287:

You are a FY2 in A&E; your current patient is in police custody. The officers ask you for a copy of the discharge summary. The patient asks you not to provide them with any of their details, however the officers insist that you must cooperate.

Rank the actions below in order of most appropriate to least appropriate:

A. Politely explain to the police that you cannot provide information without the patient's consent
B. Discuss the situation with a consultant
C. Don't give in as there are no circumstances in which you would betray your patient's confidence
D. Give a discharge summary to the patient, knowing that it might be confiscated later on
E. Give the officers a discharge summary as helping the police is in the public interest

Question 288:

It's your first week as the psychiatry FY1; you are called to a cardiac arrest. Upon arrival, you note that no-one is managing the patient's airway, despite a number of senior doctors being present. All other appropriate activities are taking place.

Rank the actions below in order of most appropriate to least appropriate:

A. Move to the patient's head and use airway adjuncts as appropriate
B. Ask the team leader why no one is managing the airway
C. Ask whether an anaesthetist is present and if not, then whether they are on their way
D. Help with chest compressions because these are easily within your comfort zone
E. Stand back so that you do not distract the arrest team leader

Question 289:

You are the urology FY1. Your registrar calls you and tells you a patient's supra-pubic catheter has fallen out and needs re-inserting. You explain that you have never done this before. He says it is simple and that no one else is free to help until the operating list finishes later.

Rank the actions below in order of most appropriate to least appropriate:

A. Ask another doctor with relevant experience to assist
B. Politely explain that you cannot perform the procedure safely and will need supervision
C. Refuse to help as you are inundated with other ward jobs
D. Read about the procedure before having a go
E. Do as you are told, but document carefully that you are acting under your registrar's instructions

Question 290:

You are the vascular surgery FY1. A patient is being treated for cellulitis of her right leg. She is improving but still requires IV antibiotics. The patient wishes to self-discharge as she is fed up with being in hospital. She is going to stay with her boyfriend who will look after her. She is fully competent. Her mother is her next of kin.

Rank the actions below in order of most appropriate to least appropriate:

A. Explain to her the risks of leaving and allow her to leave if she has understood the risks
B. Allow her to leave but advise her to see her GP for antibiotics if her cellulitis worsens
C. Allow her to leave as she is fully competent to make her own decisions
D. Telephone her boyfriend to ask him to persuade her not to leave
E. Prevent her from leaving by phoning security

Question 291:

You are working in A&E as a FY2. A non-English speaking patient attends with her 12-year-old daughter. The language barrier prevents you from obtaining a clinical history. She does not look unwell.

Rank the actions below in order of most appropriate to least appropriate:

A. Request a professional interpreter
B. Ask if there is a member of staff that speaks the same language who is willing to interpret
C. Ask the accompanying child if she is willing to act as an interpreter
D. Advise the patient to go to a GP who speaks their language
E. Refuse to see the patient on the grounds of clinical safety

Question 292:
One of the nurses asks you to have a word with one of your colleagues about his bad breath as she knows that he is one of your friends. She says that several patients have complained that they do not want to be treated by him because of this problem.

Rank the actions below in order of most appropriate to least appropriate:

A. Organise a meeting with your colleague in a quiet place and discuss this problem with him
B. Ask your colleagues if they have also noticed a problem and if they have, then have a quiet word with him
C. Ask the nurse to speak to your colleague as you do not want to risk your friendship
D. Send a note to your colleague about this problem
E. Do nothing as you do not think it is a problem

Question 293:
You see a patient with advanced lung cancer to discuss treatment options. After hearing about the risks and benefits of chemotherapy he decides to decline treatment. He clearly has capacity; his wife is shocked and asks you to ignore his wishes.

Rank the actions below in order of most appropriate to least appropriate:

A. Empathise with his wife as this must be a difficult time for them both
B. Explain to his wife that he has the right to refuse treatment
C. Document in the notes everything that has been explained during the consultation
D. Explain to the patient that you will need to take into account the views of his family
E. Ignore the wishes of the patient as no rational person declines treatment

Question 294:
You are the vascular surgery FY1 and seeing an elderly diabetic patient who has been admitted with a black toe. He asks you if he is going to lose his leg.

Rank the actions below in order of most appropriate to least appropriate:

A. Tell him that you need to take a full history and complete an examination as well as arrange some further tests. Once the test results are back a senior doctor will discuss the results with him
B. Advise him that you will need to discuss his case with your registrar before you can answer his question
C. Explain that you can't feel his foot pulses and there is a possibility he may lose his leg
D. Reassure him that everything will be okay
E. Tell him that he shouldn't worry about losing his leg as there is an expert limb fitting centre nearby

Question 295:

You have just seen a 5-year-old child in a hospital ENT clinic with a recurrent left ear discharge. You have written a prescription on a "hospital pharmacy only" prescription sheet and the patient has now left the clinic. Later, you realise that you have made an error and written a dose that is more appropriate for a large 10-year-old. Although not fatal, it is likely to make the child nauseated and diarrhoeal.

Rank the actions below in order of most appropriate to least appropriate:

A. Telephone the patient's home and leave a message telling them not to take the medicine
B. Telephone the pharmacy and tell them that you have made an error and that they should not issue the medicine
C. Speak to your consultant the next morning for advice
D. Put it down to tiredness and forget about it
E. Remove the consultation sheet from the notes so that it will be unclear who saw the child

Question 296:

You are a FY2 working in general practice. A 26-year-old woman presents with a 12-month history of abdominal pain. This has already been extensively investigated by the gastroenterology team who diagnosed her with Irritable Bowel Syndrome (IBS). Her symptoms have remained unchanged and she has no red flag features. She has done a lot of reading on the internet and thinks she has bowel or ovarian cancer. She becomes tearful and wants some blood tests, a CT scan, and another colonoscopy to be sure that there is nothing wrong.

Rank the actions below in order of most appropriate to least appropriate:

A. Reassure her and arrange to see her again in a month
B. Refer her for an ultrasound scan but agree if it is normal that no further tests will be done
C. Refer her to gastroenterology to help reassure her
D. Start her on an antidepressant
E. Request a lower gastrointestinal endoscopy

Question 297:

A patient is admitted for minor elective surgery which he has discussed with his family. Shortly before he is due to go to theatre, the patient informs you that he wants to be discharged because he has to pick up his father. There is no reason to suggest that he lacks capacity.

Rank the actions below in order of most appropriate to least appropriate:

A. Explain to the patient the risks of leaving without surgery
B. Allow the patient to leave, but request that he returns as soon as possible so that his surgery can be done at the end of the list
C. Get in touch with the patient's wife and get her to persuade the patient not to leave
D. Allow the patient to leave, but request that he sees his GP if there are any problems
E. Contact the theatre to prevent the patient from leaving

Question 298:

You are looking after a patient who has previously been treated for nasal carcinoma. Preliminary investigations are strongly suggestive of a recurrence. As you finish taking blood from a neighbouring patient, he leans across and says "Is my cancer back?".

Rank the actions below in order of most appropriate to least appropriate:

A. Inform him that you will chase up the results of his tests and speak to him yourself after
B. Explain to him that you do not have all the test results, but you will ask your registrar to speak to him as soon as you do
C. Invite him to join you and a senior nurse in a quiet room, get a colleague to hold your bleep then explore his fears at
D. Explain to him that it is likely that his cancer has come back
E. Reassure him that he will be fine as he's in good hands

Question 299:

One of your colleagues calls in sick for a night shift. That evening you see him having a meal in a restaurant. He doesn't look unwell and is eating and drinking normally. What is the most appropriate action to take?

Rank the actions below in order of most appropriate to least appropriate:

A. Ask to meet somewhere privately and discuss the situation with him. Tell his educational supervisor if he is unable to give an appropriate explanation for his actions
B. Discuss this matter with your colleagues to see if it has happened before. If it has happened before, report him to his educational supervisor
C. Tell his educational supervisor what has happened and ask them to discuss it with him
D. Ask your colleague to explain what happened in the middle of the ward in front of the nursing staff
E. Do nothing. You don't know him very well so it is nothing to do with you

Question 300:

You are the cardiology FY1. You've noticed that your patients rarely get reviewed by senior doctors even though the consultant should do at least two ward rounds per week. Yesterday, your consultant admitted that he is extremely busy with his research work and won't have time to do ward rounds in person but offered to do them remotely via phone.

Rank the actions below in order of most appropriate to least appropriate:

A. Agree to do ward rounds over the phone as long as he remains contactable throughout the week for advice.
B. Refuse politely and remind him that he is required to see all the ward patients at least twice per week in person.
C. Speak with your clinical supervisor as soon as possible for their input.
D. Report the consultant to the GMC as he is putting patient safety at risk.
E. Offer to take on some of his research work so that he has more time to do ward rounds.

ANSWERS

Q	A	Q	A	Q	A	Q	A	Q	A	Q	A
1	EACDB	26	CABDE	51	DACEB	76	DEF	101	BDCEA	126	CABED
2	ACG	27	CEBAD	52	BEH	77	EDCBA	102	DACBE	127	ECDBA
3	ACF	28	ADECB	53	ADE	78	DECBA	103	CBAED	128	ADBEC
4	DBECA	29	CAEDB	54	CEH	79	DACBE	104	DEBCA	129	ACBDE
5	DBAEC	30	AGH	55	ABDEC	80	BCEAD	105	ABCED	130	EBDAC
6	DEBCA	31	DEH	56	ABE	81	AEDBC	106	EDCBA	131	CEBAD
7	EBDCA	32	BDE	57	BEF	82	ABCDE	107	ABDCE	132	ACDEB
8	CDF	33	CABDE	58	BECDA	83	AEDBC	108	BDCAE	133	EABCD
9	ECDBA	34	ABCED	59	DCABE	84	CBDAE	109	ABECD	134	DCEBA
10	DCABE	35	AGH	60	DEACB	85	BCDEA	110	ABCDE	135	BCADE
11	BCDAE	36	EACDB	61	DEF	86	ABDEC	111	CEDAB	136	ABDEC
12	DFH	37	CBAED	62	BEADC	87	CDE	112	CEDBA	137	BCDAE
13	BADCE	38	BDEAC	63	ACBDE	88	DACEB	113	BCDAE	138	ABCED
14	AECDB	39	ACDEB	64	CEADB	89	CABDE	114	ABCED	139	EABDC
15	DECBA	40	BEDCA	65	EACDB	90	CDABE	115	CADEB	140	DCAEB
16	DBACE	41	ABCDE	66	ABEDC	91	CADBE	116	ACDEB	141	EDBCA
17	BCH	42	CFG	67	ABDEC	92	BCH	117	CDBAE	142	DCBAE
18	CDE	43	AEH	68	EDCBA	93	BAECD	118	AEDBC	143	CEABD
19	AEBDC	44	BDG	69	CABDE	94	EDBAC	119	BCDEA	144	CDEAB
20	ABE	45	BECDA	70	ADF	95	DEACB	120	CBDAE	145	CBEAD
21	EDBAC	46	DAECB	71	BEDCA	96	CGH	121	CDABE	146	BCADE
22	BDCAE	47	EDCBA	72	EDBAC	97	ACBDE	122	BEDCA	147	EDACB
23	DABCE	48	CDABE	73	EDBAC	98	ACG	123	CEDBA	148	DCBEA
24	CABDE	49	AEDCB	74	DCABE	99	AEDBC	124	DCEBA	149	ABCDE
25	BCD	50	DABCE	75	EABCD	100	EACDB	125	ECDBA	150	CEADB

Q	A	Q	A	Q	A	Q	A	Q	A	Q	A
151	DBCAE	176	DEBAC	201	ABDEC	226	DCEBA	251	CDABE	276	ACE
152	DCBEA	177	DCEBA	202	DCABE	227	BDEAC	252	BDEAC	277	BEG
153	BFH	178	CEBDA	203	CDBEA	228	CAEBD	253	ECBAD	278	CGH
154	DEF	179	ADCEB	204	CDEBA	229	BCGEG	254	CEBDA	279	ADF
155	ABD	180	CBADE	205	DAECB	230	BDH	255	DBACE	280	BAEDC
156	BDE	181	ECABD	206	EABDC	231	ABD	256	ECDAB	281	BACDE
157	ACH	182	BCDEA	207	DBAEC	232	BEG	257	BCDEA	282	CEABD
158	BDE	183	AEBDC	208	EBACD	233	AEG	258	CDEAB	283	BACED
159	BDG	184	BACDE	209	BCDEA	234	CDF	259	BCADE	284	CEBDA
160	BDE	185	ACDBE	210	BDECA	235	BDH	260	DEF	285	ADBCE
161	CGH	186	ABCED	211	CBAED	236	CDH	261	ADG	286	ACBDE
162	DFG	187	DCEAB	212	ACBED	237	BEG	262	ADG	287	ABECD
163	BEF	188	CDBAE	213	BECAD	238	BFG	263	BCD	288	BCDEA
164	DEG	189	DECAB	214	ECBAD	239	BDG	264	ABF	289	BAECD
165	BCD	190	EBACD	215	ECBDA	240	BEF	265	ADH	290	CABED
166	ABF	191	EBCDA	216	BDCEA	241	BCE	266	AGH	291	BACDE
167	CGH	192	ADECB	217	BEDAC	242	ADE	267	CFH	292	DBAEC
168	BFG	193	CBDAE	218	EBACD	243	CDF	268	CDE	293	BACDE
169	CFH	194	CEABD	219	DEACB	244	BEG	269	CDE	294	ABCDE
170	ADE	195	DCABE	220	BEACD	245	ABG	270	BFH	295	BACDE
171	CDG	196	DACBE	221	DEBAC	246	BEG	271	AGH	296	ABCED
172	ABD	197	CBDAE	222	BDF	247	BCG	272	BDE	297	DBAEC
173	ABF	198	DCBEA	223	AEG	248	BDH	273	CGH	298	BACDE
174	BDG	199	DABCE	224	BGH	249	CEF	274	AEF	299	ACEBD
175	ADECB	200	DECAB	225	BEG	250	AEBCD	275	ABD	300	BCDEA

WORKED ANSWERS

Question 1: EACDB

It is important to maintain a good working relationship with the nursing staff as their help can be vital when you are very busy. E is the best course of action as it solves the current situation and prevents it from reoccurring in the future, as well as allowing you to maintain a good working relationship. Whilst A is technically true, it does not attempt to address the current situation and is unlikely to help the working relationship, so it is the next best option. C is not ideal as it does not solve the current situation and will not help to promote a good working relationship with the nursing staff, even though the complaint is unlikely to go any further. D is a highly antagonistic and inappropriate course of action that does not help the situation. However, it is still better than B which is completely unacceptable as it could directly harm patients and be very dangerous. Treating patients should always be the main priority.

Question 2: ACG

There will be times when you feel tired and unable to perform your best at your job, however, in this situation, your friend poses an infection risk to the patients from her vomiting. Even though it would be tempting to give her symptomatic relief so she can feel better and help you, this would not address the fact that she should not be in work whilst potentially infectious. Therefore, D is wrong. B and F would be unhelpful to the situation. E is inappropriate as taking hospital supplies may affect the supply available for patients. Ultimately, the best courses of action for the patients are A and G, which may mean more work for you but will avoid any potential harm to the patient. C is the next best option as it will allow your colleague to feel better and help you with the busy ward. It may also be a better option to expose the patients to a small risk of infection with a doctor who is feeling better after taking some paracetamol, rather than leaving the ward short staffed.

Question 3: ACF

It would always be advisable to speak to the first doctor to find out why they refused to sign the prescription (A). Since the nurse has expressed concerns about the patient, it would be wise to assess them (C) to see if they need the prescription urgently. It is also sensible to advise the nurse to discuss her concerns with the doctor in the future to prevent this situation reoccurring. Maintaining communication will allow such problems to be solved more directly.

Question 4: DBECA

Maintaining confidentiality is paramount for the care and trust of patients in the health service as well as their privacy. Taking a list home with confidential patient information is against most trusts' policies as the security of these lists in people's homes is not assured. Therefore, to inform your colleague that they should not risk breaking patient's confidentiality is the best answer, (D) as it instantly deals with the problem. Asking for more confidential waste bins (B) may deal with the problem eventually, but does not fix the immediate problem. Speaking to your consultant (E) again would fix the problem but could damage your working relationship with your colleague. C may do nothing to solve the problem, or even alert your colleague that you are noticing what they are doing. A is absolutely the wrong thing to do as it does nothing to reduce the risk of breaking patient confidentiality.

Question 5: DBAEC

As an NHS doctor, your main concern should be your patients. It is inappropriate for you to compromise on their care to satisfy your consultant when what they are asking is unreasonable. The best answer is D, to speak to them and explain this as it is likely to solve the situation. The next best option is B, to speak to other consultants as they may be able to offer you advice. The remaining answers are all the wrong things to do, but A is the least wrong because it will allow the private patient to be seen, but you would have to be careful as you may not be covered by the hospital to treat patients after your shift has ended. Clerking the patient quickly will not solve the situation (E) as the consultant is likely to ask again, and this may be detrimental to your NHS patients. Ignoring the message (C) is the worst thing to do since the consultant may assume that the work has been done and may harm the private patient.

Question 6: DEBCA

Performing the drain incorrectly could cause the patient more harm than good, so it is the worst option (A), and it is only slightly better to do this with guidance (C). Bleeping the more experienced FY2 is the next best option as it will mean someone more senior is likely to be able to perform the drain competently (B), however, this may delay the procedure. Refusing (E) to do the drain is correct as it could harm the patient but it is appropriate to offer to help (D) as taking the timings in a cardiac arrest is imperative.

Question 7: EBDCA

Calling your colleague and asking where they are is the best option (E), as they may be delayed elsewhere in the hospital such that you can find them to hand over the jobs. Calling to see if they are sick (B) is the next best option as it will hopefully allow for alternative cover to be made. Handing over to another doctor (D) is acceptable as it will ensure someone is aware of the jobs, but is less than ideal because it may add to this doctor's workload. Waiting for your colleague to arrive (C) is inappropriate as you have been working all day and are likely to be tired, which may impact on your patients. Leaving a written handover (A) is the worst thing to do as it may never get seen if your colleague is not coming in and could cause significant patient harm.

Question 8: CDF

C, D and F are the three best options as you should not perform a procedure unsupervised until you are fully competent. It is appropriate to offer an alternative (C) temporary contraception and try to find out how long the consultant will be (D) so you can inform the patient of the waiting time. Asking another senior (F) to supervise you performing the implant is also suitable as it allows the patient to leave with the implant in place. Options A and H are incorrect because it would be wrong to perform the procedure if you are not competent. B is wrong as you do not know when the consultant will return and may not have time to supervise when they return. Option E puts an unfair choice on the patient as she is obviously keen to leave and might not be aware that you are not competent at the procedure. F is a safe option as you are not performing the procedure without being competent, but will leave the patient without contraception for the interim which is why it is not one of the three best options.

Question 9: ECDBA

Sustaining a needle stick is a stressful experience which should be dealt with as quickly as possible. E is the best option as it should minimise the exposure to the patient's blood and is standard protocol. Reporting to occupational health is also important, (C) as you will be able to obtain post-exposure prophylaxis and allow the department to arrange further blood tests for yourself and the patient. D is appropriate but is not as much of a high-priority as minimising the risk to yourself. Carrying on with the operation is inappropriate because it does not reduce the immediate risk, especially as your consultant says they are able to finish the operation alone. A is very inappropriate since it would be unethical to test a patient's blood for HIV status without consent.

Question 10: DCABE

D is the best option because the patient states that they have difficulty obtaining GP appointments, so this may delay them receiving the correct antibiotics. Therefore, they can collect a prescription from you as they are under the hospital for their upcoming surgery. Asking the patient to attend their local A&E (C) will mean they get quick treatment for their UTI but is not the best option as they may have to wait to be seen, whereas you can sort the problem quickly. A is not ideal since the patient has already explained that they struggle to get GP appointments so they may have a long delay before they can receive their antibiotics. B is worse than A because the letter will take even longer than the patient booking an appointment themselves. E is the worst option as a simple UTI is not severe enough to warrant cancelling their operation, and may cause them harm.

Question 11: BCDAE

The best thing to do in this situation is to ask for help from someone more senior. The first port of call should be your FY2 (B) who may have more luck with establishing venous access or help you decide that it is okay to switch the patient to other treatment not requiring venous access. Although not ideal for them, calling the anaesthetists (C) would be the next best option as it is likely that the patient needs the fluids and antibiotics, and they are often more experienced at difficult cannulation. When the first two options have failed, D would be the best alternative choice as it will at least provide the patient with some antibiotics even if they are not as good as the IV form. Leaving the day team to review is potentially harmful to the patient (A), so is inappropriate and inferior to asking for help to sort a solution. E is the worst option as it goes directly against the patient's wishes and you should always ask for help first.

Question 12: DFH

The best options are D, F and H as they provide the student with an opportunity to correct his work and admit his mistake. F is the best first action, as although it is unlikely, it may be that the patient the student saw simply resembled yours. D and H are also appropriate as the student may not have been aware that what he was doing would go against GMC guidance on honesty and plagiarism, and this gives him another opportunity to do the case report properly without escalating it further. Option A is unnecessary at this stage and may result in a formal warning or could even prevent the student from progressing through medical school. B is inappropriate as it is not okay for the student to continue to copy others' work and it is important to ascertain whether he knew what he was doing was wrong. If it was a misunderstanding, then it can simply be resolved, and as a doctor, you are part of the team for educating him on the qualities expected, so to do nothing would be neglecting your duties in this sense. Asking the consultant (C) what they think or reading the GMC guidelines (E) about plagiarism is unhelpful because it will only confirm what you know to be true. Informing the consultant (G) is not necessary at this stage and may be avoided by first attempting the other more appropriate steps.

Question 13: BADCE

B is the most appropriate response because it could immediately resolve the situation if you are mistaken. A is the next best option as your senior may be able to discuss this with the healthcare assistant and solve the problem without escalating it in a way that could prevent a disproportional response. D is better than C because you could be wrong and they may be taking the medicines for a patient. Informing personnel before you are sure what is going on may prevent the healthcare assistant from potentially working with patients and would likely damage your working relationship. E is the worst option as it potentially puts patients at risk and does not attempt to resolve the situation.

Question 14: AECDB

A is the best thing to do as it prevents you from lying to the patient. It is better than E because it involves senior colleagues to discuss the matter with the patient. C is a good thing to do as it will give the patient the opportunity to ask questions in a private setting, but leaving your bleep may compromise the care of other patients. D is not ideal as the diagnosis has not been confirmed and does not allow him the chance to have a relative with him to receive the bad news. B is the worst option since it means lying to the patient and will likely damage his trust in you if the results come back indicating that he does have cancer.

Question 15: DECBA

Patient care is the absolute priority in this question and the best way to ensure their safety while maintaining a good relationship with your colleague is D. E and C will likely harm your working relationship but are the next best options to protect your patients, with E being the better option as your consultant may be able to help your colleague and ensure the safety of your patients without any formal action occurring. B is inappropriate as it is unfair to ask the nurses to go easy on your colleague and is likely to put more pressure on other doctors. However, B is better than A which could mean the situation continues and patient care is at risk.

Question 16: DBACE

Exploring the patient's concerns (D) is the best thing to do as it may elucidate why the patient is hesitant to allow your colleague to perform the procedure. Ultimately, if the patient does not want your registrar to treat him, you should tell your colleague (B) so that the patient is not treated against his wishes. This may save your colleague some embarrassment. GMC guidance states that the patient is the primary concern with their views being taken into account, so even if you personally disagree with the patient's views, it should not be allowed to affect your working relationship. Therefore, option A is the next best option. C is the first wrong option, as it does not respect the patient's choice. E is the worst thing to do as it may harm the patient and does not respect his views.

Question 17: BCH

Speaking to a senior (B) and the safeguarding team (H) is always advised in cases of domestic violence since it keeps them informed of the situation. It also allows them to advise you on the best course of action. Offering the patient support (C) will alert the patient to her options available and may encourage her to seek help in the future. Informing her partner (A) is a very bad idea as it is unlikely to not solve the situation and could even make it worse, encouraging more violence to your patient or even yourself. Contacting the GP (D) is passing the duty of care of this patient to another doctor who may be unaware of the situation, and it is not guaranteed that your patient will be as forthcoming with them as they have been with you. Informing the police (E) is not ideal because the patient does not want any further action at this stage and is unlikely to make a statement against her partner. Doing nothing (F) without consulting a senior or the appropriate department for advice is the wrong thing to do. Calling the partner (G) is also wrong as it may alert him to your suspicions and is unlikely to solve the situation.

Question 18: CDE

GMC guidance states to involve patients in decisions about their treatment and that you must respect a competent patients' choice to refuse treatment even if you disagree with them. However, in the case of children, you should ideally involve the child in a way that is appropriate to their maturity and age, unless it is an emergency when it is necessary to save their life. So, ultimately, giving the blood (C) is the right thing to do for this child, but you would ideally explain to the parents (E) why their son needs the blood in the hope they will consent to the treatment. You should always involve your seniors (D) as they may be more experienced in similar situations and be able to help. All of the other options are inappropriate because treating the boy without the blood (A and H) is likely to result in grave consequences for him and is against GMC guidance for this exceptional circumstance. Calling the chaplain (B) is likely to delay the transfusion and may not even be successful. However, it may be helpful to designate a family point of contact for the future as relations with them could be difficult after acting against their wishes. Scaring the parents (F) is an unfair method and will likely reduce their trust in you, making them even less likely to consent. Asking the parents about their son's wishes (G) is not actually relevant as GMC guidance states that in emergency situations involving a child, the wishes of the parents can be overruled if the treatment is necessary to save the child's life or prevent deterioration in health. It could also delay the urgently needed treatment.

Question 19: AEBDC

Whilst it is important for all members to behave professionally whilst working, it is okay for doctors to enjoy themselves and have personal lives so long as it does not impact on patient care. In this case, the best option is to not divulge any personal information (A) and allow your friend to respond herself. Informing your friend (E) is the next best thing as it will allow her to respond how she likes. The registrar is unlikely to have spoken to you as her friend if he does not want you to tell her. The remaining options are inappropriate as walking away (B) is an overreaction to the situation since there does not seem to be any inappropriate behaviour taking place at present. Telling your consultant (D) is unprofessional as it involves them unnecessarily in the social situation and could create tension in your team. Giving away your friend's phone number (C) and revealing personal information on her behalf is the wrong thing to do as it puts her in a difficult situation where she may not wish to be involved. This could create working tensions in the team, with your friend not having had the opportunity to talk to the registrar first.

Question 20: ABE

This question highlights the difficulties of maintaining patient confidentiality and their safety when they are contradictory. The best options, B, A, and E will all hopefully stop this gentleman from driving and putting himself and others at risk. Informing his wife (D) is a breach of confidentiality and involving the police at this stage (F) is not ideal until reasonable attempts have been made to stop him from driving whilst still drinking. Informing the DVLA (A) may be necessary as he is putting himself, and others at risk- thus a breach of confidentiality may be justified in this case. C is very inappropriate as he may cause harm to himself or others while he is still drinking and driving in the meantime, even if he successfully undertakes a detox.

Question 21: EDBAC

In certain specialities such as gynaecology and urology, patients may often refuse to see doctors due to their gender; wishes you must respect as far as possible. In this instance, it is difficult to determine whether the presentation is life-threatening, but either way, you must aim to respect the patients' request as much as possible. As the patient has the capacity and has specifically requested for you not to examine her, it would be wrong to do so against her will (C). In an emergency situation where it is not possible to obtain consent, however, it would be prudent to proceed without this, acting in the patient's best interests (A). It may be possible to wait for a female doctor (B), and if so, this is preferred to only taking a history. The best thing to do would be to offer a compromise (E) as this will hopefully provide a quick and easy solution to the problem, causing the minimal disruption to other doctors and giving the patient the examination she needs. The next best thing to do is to explain the urgency of the situation, (D) which may then reassure the patient that you are acting in their best interests and could convince them to allow you to do the examination. Waiting for another doctor (B) whilst respecting the patient's wishes is a neutral response in this situation as it may allow the patient to put themselves unknowingly at risk since they might not understand the urgency of the situation.

Question 22: BDCAE

The best thing to do in the face of dissatisfied patients and their families is to explore their concerns (B) and try to rectify the situation at the time if possible. If this fails, informing the team (D) is appropriate as it could prepare them for a formal complaint and allow for a discussion about any concerns in advance. This may alleviate the situation by talking to the relative and explaining any issues. Suggesting the relative speaks to another department (C) is not a bad response but is not as good as trying to deal with the situation directly where there may just be a misunderstanding. (A) Is the first wrong answer because it is not right to discourage patients and their families from expressing their concerns, but is still better than you, yourself complaining (E) and encouraging others to do so.

Question 23: DABCE

While looking after private patients when you are working an NHS shift is not part of your normal responsibilities, it would be wrong not to help in an urgent situation. Therefore, the best thing to do is assess the situation for its urgency (D) relative to your other jobs and proceed from there. The next best thing to do is help with the current problem (A) but make it clear you will not always be able to do so as it could interfere with your work in a way that harms your other patients. Enquiring about who is available (B) is the next best choice because it could prevent problems in the future. However, this does not address the current situation. Asking for payment (C) when you are working on NHS time is inappropriate even with a private patient, but is better than refusing to help altogether (E) as this may significantly harm the patient in question.

Question 24: CABDE

There are various fundamental skills that all junior doctors must be able to undertake such as cannulation, venepuncture, and ABGs. Ideally, the issue would have been raised earlier, but in this instance, the best thing to do would be to help your colleague (C) learn so it can solve their inability to do so quickly. Advising them to seek senior guidance (A) is the next best option because it will help them learn the skill. These direct solutions are better than emailing their advisor (B) as they are likely to know you have raised this issue and will wonder why you did not approach them first. As you are able to do the ABGs, there is no immediate risk to patient safety, so the second worse option is to allow them to come to you (D). However, this would be better than embarrassing them in front of a patient (E) which is unprofessional and will likely damage your working relationship.

Question 25: BCD

In this scenario, it would be prudent to offer advice about safe sex (D) as this patient has been presented with a sexually transmitted disease. As he has engaged in unprotected sexual activity with another man, it would also be advisable to offer him an HIV test (B) and to inform his partner so she can be tested. This is not mandatory (E), however, and whilst it would be advised for him to tell his girlfriend (A) and his male partner (H), he does not have to and you are not required to tell either of them or his GP (F). It is inappropriate to judge this patient's relationship and offer counselling (G) unless he asks for it.

Question 26: CABDE

It is imperative that you do not miss non-accidental injuries, especially in children and other vulnerable groups. The best thing to do would be to document the boy's claims (C) and ask more questions to investigate them fully. The next best thing would be to examine the boy (A) and look for any signs to support his accusations (A). However, it makes no mention of documentation, which is very important in this case as if it progresses further, your information is likely to provide evidence. Asking the father about the claims (B) before gathering more information could antagonise him but would need to be undertaken before escalating the claims. Calling the police (D) as an FY1 without first talking to your seniors would not be advised, however, it would be preferable to ignoring the claims (E) as this risks leaving the child in a potentially abusive situation.

Question 27: CEBAD

Whilst a DNACPR order is a medical decision, it is important to communicate this decision to the patient and their family. As it is not an immediate problem, it would be best to discuss this with the patient first (C) who may then want to involve their family. Discussing this with your seniors would be appropriate (E) as they may have experienced similar situations previously and could potentially advise you. The next option (B) is a neutral one as it is probably not a discussion you should engage in alone as an FY1. Apologising for other doctors is the first wrong option (A) because there may have been reasons for this misunderstanding and you do not know what might have been communicated and why. The worst thing to do would be to ignore the order (D) as it is relevant regardless of whether the patient is informed, and it would be inappropriate for you, as an FY1, to ignore the order without senior involvement.

Question 28: ADECB

Removing hospital equipment without permission, even for the benefit of your own medical studies, is not acceptable under any circumstances and constitutes theft. The best option is to ask him to return the equipment (A), followed by the threat of reporting him if he continues to do so (D). Failing this, you would have to tell the theatre manager (E) so that they know about the missing items and can restock the theatres appropriately. Reporting him to a supervisor (C) is extreme before exhausting other options, but the worst answer is to do nothing (B), because as an FY1, he is unlikely to be undertaking any surgery without supervision. Therefore, the need to practise does not supersede the theft taking place.

Question 29: CAEDB

When consenting a patient, the guidance from the GMC is that the doctor performing the operation should be the one to obtain consent, but they can ask another doctor to do this as long as they have sufficient knowledge about the operation and the risk it carries. The best option, in this case, is then C. As an FY1, you are unlikely to have the experience required to consent the patient. The next choice would be to find another doctor (A) with the sufficient experience so as not to delay the morning list. However, this is not the best answer as it may take them away from their current tasks. Seeking advice (E) shows you do not have the knowledge required and so is the first wrong answer, but is better than the final options of taking the consent without any help at all. Of the two, doing the consent immediately is better (D) as it may allow for any problems with the consent to be sorted more quickly and prevent any delay to the morning list (B).

Question 30: AGH

There will often be times when you are working when you feel tired and hungry. You must not allow these to impact on patient safety, so the best option here is to explain this to the nurse (A) and offer to do the prescriptions later (G) since making mistakes could be very harmful. It would also be right to ask about the urgency (H) to ensure a patient is not going without any needed medicine before you go on a break. It would be wrong to be unhelpful (B) and offer no solution, or pass the job on to someone else (C) if it is your responsibility. Nevertheless, doing these when you could make mistakes (D), (F) or asking the nurse to do the prescription (E) are also wrong answers.

Question 31: DEH

Basic clinical skills such as cannulation and venepuncture are crucial for an FY1 to be competent enough to pass their foundation year. The best solutions will be to practise in the hope you will improve and boost your confidence, whether on patients who need them (D) or in the laboratory (H). Asking a senior to supervise (E) is also a good option as they may be able to identify any problems in your techniques. It would be wrong to practise on patients who do not need such procedures (G). Equally, avoiding patients who need them (B), or constantly asking your colleagues for help (A) (F) may unfairly add to their workload. Changing careers (C) would be too dramatic for skills that can be learned with practice.

Question 32: BDE

Confusion is a common problem and has many causes. Often, the patients are delirious and may become disruptive on the ward, or even threatening and abusive to staff. In this situation, the best thing to do would be to attempt to calm the patient (B) and ask the nurses (E) or security (D) if necessary. It would be wrong to allow the patient to leave (A) or move the patient to another ward (H) when they are clearly acutely unwell. There is no evidence at this stage of a psychiatric problem (C), so a review is inappropriate at this stage. Sedating the patient (F) should be a last resort and bleeping the surgeon (G) will not solve the immediate problem.

Question 33: CABDE

This question tests your ability to balance the areas of consent and confidentiality, with the added difficulty of it concerning a minor. It is never wrong to act in the patients' best interests, which in this situation involves giving her the treatment. As she is intelligent, she can consent for herself, but it would be best to explore her concerns (C) so that she may be encouraged to involve her parents, especially as she is engaging in sexual activity. If she still refuses, the next best thing would be to give her the treatment (A) as it is in her greatest interests. The remaining answers are the wrong things to do because you do not have to inform her parents if she does not wish you to, and is competent to consent for herself. The least bad is B, as it encourages her to tell her parents herself. Followed by informing them yourself (D), which is still better than refusing her the treatment altogether (E) which is clearly not in her best interests.

Question 34: ABCED

This scenario represents a common occurrence in many busy hospitals. It is a radiologist's job to ensure that patients' investigations using radiation are justified. Therefore, they are correct to ask for more information if they are not satisfied with that provided. The best thing to do in this scenario would be to contact your registrar (A) as they may know the information required and could save you from having to bother your consultant while he is busy in surgery (B). Asking the radiologists to go straight to your consultant (C) is passing the responsibility and adds to their workload, so you should try to help first. It would be wrong to ignore the situation (E), but even worse to give potentially incorrect information (D) as this may result in the scan being done for the wrong reasons.

Question 35: AGH
Whilst all doctors in their junior years should receive ample support and teaching from their seniors, there will often be a discrepancy between attachments due to the differing level seniors available and how busy the firm is. You should seek out teaching opportunities but not at the expense of caring for your patients or your own personal life. The best options would be to approach your consultant (A) or your educational supervisor (G) as they might be able to help with the rota and offer you teaching opportunities. Failing this, checking your contract is important (H) if you are consistently working longer than your contracted hours to ensure that you are paid accordingly. It would be wrong to neglect your patients (B) (D) in order to make sure you are being fairly treated before asking for help, as this could harm your patients. Equally to struggle on (C) organising your own teaching (E) as this should be provided for you. Taking time off (F) should be avoided as this could leave the rota even further stretched and may affect patient care.

Question 36: EACDB
Patients are often very grateful for the care they receive during their stays in hospital and may often want to thank you and other members of the team for looking after them. You are allowed to accept gifts from patients as long as they are proportional to the level of treatment you provided. For example, receiving a box of chocolates for being their ward doctor is okay, but taking a large sum of money would not be. When accepting recurring gifts, you should be more discerning and use your judgement and explore the reasons for which the gift was given. In this instance, accepting the gift but enquiring the reasons for it (E) would be the best response as you may find the patient feels obliged to do so, to whom you can allay the concerns of without causing offence. Failing this, you should ask your seniors to decline the gift (A) as they may be more experienced with refusing such gifts without causing offence and harming your relationship with the patient. Accepting the gift but explaining that you will share it (C) is a neutral option since it does not explore the reasons for the gift, but affirms that you are not just accepting a reward for yourself for their treatment. It is wrong to refuse but then accept if they insist (D), but even more so to continually accept the gifts (B) without question.

Question 37: CBAED
In this unfortunate situation, the best thing to do is to accept the responsibility for your error and apologise (C), it would then be appropriate to arrange to meet your supervisor (B) to discuss the problems. Recording the error (A) is a neutral response as it is confined to your personal improvement and does nothing to rectify the problems with the long hours. It would be wrong to blame the long hours (E) without accepting the responsibility, but better than asking the nurse to go against the guidelines and not report the error (D).

Question 38: BDEAC
When managing any patient, the first priority should be to assess them to check they are well and do not need any immediate treatment (B). The next best thing to do would be to consult the trust guidelines (D) as there will often be guidance on how to proceed. Bleeping the medical registrar is the next appropriate thing to do (E) but is not the best as it adds to what will probably be a considerable workload, when you may be able to manage the patient yourself. Using the internet is risky (A) as you can never be sure of the validity of unofficial online resources, but it is better than blindly prescribing a medicine you think may help (C), which could harm the patient.

Question 39: ACDEB

As job changeover between foundation jobs occurs so often, it is important that you do your best to ensure a smooth transition between rotations by not leaving any outstanding work and a clear handover to your successor. Considering the difficulties you faced, the best thing to do would be to discuss these with your supervisor (A) as they may be in a position to change things such that the next doctor is more supported and provides a better induction. Failing this, the next best option would be to make a clear list (C) so that your successor is well informed with useful information that will hopefully relieve some of the strain. Leaving your contact details (D) is a neutral response as it may mean you are inundated with calls for help, impacting on your own work (E), but it would be worse to allow your own work and patients to suffer by taking time off your next rotation (B) to help.

Question 40: BEDCA

This is a tricky situation where you have conflicting accounts from a patient and a nurse, but failing to receive the medicine could be putting the patient at risk so it must be addressed. Assessing the patient for their memory ability (B) is the best thing to do to ensure that the patient is simply not remembering the events, which is possible considering their disease. The next best choice would be to ask the ward sister to get involved (E) as she may have more information and will be more experienced to help. Filing a report (D) is the next option as it would be better to approach the nurse in question or the ward sister, as with option C, which is premature without further investigating the matter first. Changing the medications (A) does not address the current and potential future issues with either the nurse's failure or patient's current non-compliance in the future. This may cause unnecessary risk to the patient.

Question 41: ABCDE

In such a situation where a doctor's ability to detect key details about the state of a patient is in question, it is also a question of patient safety and cannot be ignored. Trying to cover for your registrar by examining the patients after him (E) will take significant time and will not solve the problem, making it the worst option. Whilst approaching the registrar directly is a good thing to do, offering to teach him (D) is likely to cause offence and not help the situation. Informing the head of the department (C) is escalating prematurely when you could speak to you consultant first which is the best option (A). But if this fails again, contacting your supervisor is the next best thing to do (B).

Question 42: CFG

The patient may have had a dangerous overdose of the drug, so assessing them is the top priority (C). Unfortunately, you will need to report this incident (F) as it would be wrong for you to cover clinical errors, so you must also make a formal report (G) on whatever system your hospital uses. Seeing the patient but avoiding documenting this (A) would also be wrong, as well as telling them not to take their next dose (D). This could be more harmful than good and also covers up the mistake. Escalating the matter to have the nurse removed (B) is inappropriate because the nurse does not pose an immediate threat to other patients as she has owned up to the mistake, and this may leave the ward short staffed. Ignoring the situation (E), or just writing in their notes (H) are also inappropriate choices because it could harm the patient.

Question 52: BEH
Being very busy as a first-year doctor, you may often forget to do some things throughout your long day and only realise on your way home. It may occasionally be suitable to leave the task until you return, but in this case, it could potentially cause damage to patient care so you should attempt to rectify the problem. Therefore, the best options are B, E, and H. You should always try and maintain a work-life balance so it would be wrong to set aside your personal life (C) (D) unless there is an immediate risk to your patients' safety. It would be wrong to neglect the task until the morning (A) (G) because doing so could compromise the patient's care. Additionally, it is inappropriate to ask nurses to give medicine without a prescription even prospectively.

Question 53: ADE
There will often be times where you and members of your team are struggling to balance your normal routine daily tasks with those required to help with career progression. It is important to be sympathetic and helpful during these times, but never at the expense of patient safety. In this case, it would be inappropriate for you to accept the bleep, so the best options are those that do this (A), (D), and (E). Accepting the bleep but asking for advice (B), (F), (G), (H) for other team members is still inappropriate regardless of who you ask advice from, as in an emergency, for example, this may delay treatment which could compromise patient care. It is also unnecessary to ask for consultant advice (C) at this stage when you can sort the issue yourself.

Question 54: CEH
Dealing with children and consent is a difficult issue and especially more so when it concerns sexual activity and those approaching the age of consent. GMC guidance states that even for underage people, if it is in their best interests to receive the contraception, and are likely to otherwise continue having sex without it, you should prescribe it (H). It is also important to ask about their relationship (C) to ensure it is consensual. You should encourage these young people to tell their parents (E), but they do not have to, so D and G are wrong. Refusing to prescribe would not be in this patient's best interests (A), nor is it necessary to inform the police (B) or social services (F), though you may need to consider this in a younger patient, or if you suspect some sort of abuse.

Question 55: ABDEC
GMC guidance about forming a relationship with patients dictates that it is inappropriate to have a relationship with any vulnerable patients, such as with this patient. So, the best option is to explain this (A), or failing that, allow them to contact you at work to ensure you maintain a professional relationship (B) and do not cause offence. Informing a consultant is also a good thing to do because they may have experience of similar situations and be able to offer advice. Contacting the patient would be the wrong thing to do but it would be worse to do it immediately (C), rather than waiting until they are less vulnerable (E).

Question 56: ABE
When considering whether to accept any gift from a patient, it is imperative to contemplate its appropriateness to the care provided. In this scenario, the gift is obviously overly generous for the care provided and so it should be refused (B), explaining that it is not necessary (A). It would also be prudent to enquire about the reasons for giving the gift (E) as it may reveal that the patient feels beholden to the staff and worried about causing offence. Any answers accepting the gift, regardless of with whom you offer to share it with are wrong (C), (D), (E), (G). In this instance, the gift is over proportional to the service given. Neither is it appropriate for your consultant to accept the gift on your behalf.

Question 57: BEF

This is a difficult situation. When dealing with patients who have trouble understanding their medicine routines, it is very important to be clear and clarify any misunderstandings (B). Endocrine patients can be on a large cocktail of drugs which get added over a long period of time. Hence, it's important to review the drug chart and see if there are drugs that could be consolidated into a single dose or stopped. Since you're a FY1, you should always check complex decisions like this with a senior doctor before (E). The other option is to explore alternative means of support for the patient to help them with their medications (F). [Options with the word 'explore' are always a good bet if you're stuck!]

Asking their GP to go through their medications (D) is not ideal as the GP may not have a good working knowledge of specialist endocrine medicine and it also defers the job to another healthcare professional where you could solve the problem directly. Worse still would be to just tell the patient to book an appointment with their GP without giving the GP any information (A). Falsely reassuring the patient to alter their medication schedule (C) or stopping them yourself without senior input (H) is not a good idea as it might lead to harming the patient. There is not information here to conclude that a carer is necessary (G) and arranging one without exploring the issue further would be presumptuous.

Question 58: BECDA

It is important that you understand the indications for any sort of investigations, not only for the best interests of the patient, but to be able to defend yourself against any legal action that may follow. If you are unsure, it would be best to discuss this again with the consultant (B) as they may have misunderstood some details about the patient. Asking another more senior doctor (E) would be the next best option, but is not as good because of the fact that it will take more time to explain all of the clinical details and may cause issues with the consultant for not asking them directly.

Question 59: DCABE

This is an unfortunate situation, as it is very important to deal with all needle stick injuries as soon as possible. By acting quickly, you are more likely to prevent harm and reduce the chances of contraction of blood-borne diseases. Protecting patients from any harm is the main priority so the assistant should refrain from any further procedures (D) since they now constitute high-risk until they have been cleared from infections. She should then seek advice (C), followed by contacting the patient involved (A). They will hopefully be willing to provide a blood sample which can be tested, but guidance states that someone external to the situation should do this so they do not feel unduly pressured. Acting to prevent infection (B) would have been a very good option at the time but is now unlikely to help. It is wrong to report her to the ward sister (E) as no patient has been put in harm's way.

Question 60: DEACB

If possible, it is best to maintain a good relationship with the families of patients, but there may come times where this is difficult. It is imperative that you act in the patient's best interests and protect their autonomy as much as possible, so the best answer is D. Even if you do not agree with the patient, you should respect their wishes assuming they have the capacity to make their own medical decisions. Asking for senior help (E) is always a good option, but in this case, it comes after (D) because it would be better to respect the patient's autonomy first. Performing a memory assessment (A) is a neutral response because you have already judged her to be competent, but is unlikely to cause any harm and may mean you have more information to give the family to support your decision. It is wrong to treat a patient against their will, so the least bad of the two remaining options is C as it respects their autonomy more than B, which ignores it completely.

Question 61: DEF

This question tests whether you recognise the need to protect patient's confidential information as well as being helpful with professional relationships between patients and their families. It is imperative that you ask for the patient's consent (D). Asking the nurses involved with the patient's care (F) is a good idea as they will probably have more of the clinical information and may be aware of any family situation that would prevent you imparting this information. As you do not know them, it is possible that you won't know whether the patient is happy for this relative to have their information shared. Explaining the situation (E) is the final correct answer, as you should do your best even when covering a shift to help with relative questions. Most people will be more understanding if you are honest and explain the situation. Your normal consultant is unlikely to have any more information about this patient (A). Telling the patient to wait for their normal team (B) is handing over responsibility and does not deal with the relative's immediate concerns. Even when covering a shift, you have a duty of care to the patients and their relatives. Contacting the normal team (C) when they are not working is inappropriate if the situation is not urgent, as with this. Telling the relative everything you know (G) without first checking with the patient is just as wrong as refusing to tell them anything (H).

Question 62: BEADC

It is important to maintain a professional relationship with your patients such that you have a good rapport but are not overly friendly and inappropriate. Patients may find it hard to reject any advances from you to establish a relationship outside work, so you must be sensitive towards this. GMC guidance states that you should not have any sort of extra relationship with a current patient, so the best option in this scenario is to explain this (B). You can then ask for advice (E) from another GP who will be experienced enough to give guidance on how to handle the situation. Offering to contact them (A) is not an ideal response since they are still currently under your care, and this may encourage the patient to change doctors in order to stay in contact. It would be wrong to offer to contact the patient (D), but still worse to lie to the patient (C) saying that you will contact them and then not do so.

Question 63: ACBDE

With an increasingly busy NHS, you will always be under pressure to send patients home as soon as possible. It is very important, however, that you do not compromise patient care for the sake of bed space and send unwell patients home, so this is the worst option (E). If you are worried, the best option would be to ask your consultant (A) to reassess the patient, as they will already be familiar with the patient from the ward round. Failing this, the next best decision would be to ask your registrar (C) as they will have sufficient experience, but this is less appropriate than the consultant. Asking another team's consultant (B) is wrong since they are unlikely to be familiar with this particular patient, and it may come across as though you are undermining your consultant. Keeping the patient in without assessing them (D) is also wrong, but is better than letting a potentially unwell patient go home (E).

Question 64: CEABD

This is a very difficult situation where you have to balance the potential harm to patients against the damage to your working relationship that addressing it could cause. In this case, the wrong treatment could have devastating consequences to your patients if a time comes where you are unable to check them. Dealing with the issue directly by speaking to the SHO in question (C) will allow the SHO to explain their rationale behind their advice (you may be mistaken or they could be following other guidelines). The next best option is to talk to your consultant (E), as this directly deal with the issue. However, it is less ideal than speaking to them directly which is likely to damage your professional relationship. Sharing your concerns with your supervisor (A) is appropriate but will not deal with the issue as quickly, and could allow patients to come to harm in the meantime. Although you should do everything to prevent patients coming to harm, continuing to check up on your colleague (B) is not going to improve the system – merely stop it from getting worse. It also doesn't address the issue directly and risks you burning out. Talking to the nurses (D) may provide more evidence for your concerns but is more likely to cause issues than help with how to proceed.

Question 65: EACDB

In this increasingly internet-dominated age, patients have greater access to online resources for medical information, the validity of which will vary from site to site. When a patient reads a bit of information that is inaccurate, such as may have occurred in this case, it presents a challenge where the best thing to do is explore their concerns and explain why they do not need a particular medicine (E) and that it may do them harm. You should also inform them that they can ask for a second opinion (A) if they are still anxious. Refusing the medication (C) without any sort of explanation is not a good thing to do, but is better than giving it to a patient who does not need it. Of the remaining options, at least reviewing soon after (D) will hopefully allow you to prevent any serious harm taking place rather than giving into the patient altogether (B).

Question 66: ABEDC

This is a difficult situation where you are not sure of the patient's capacity to consent for medical treatment. The best thing to do would be to assess their cognition (A) so you can determine this, although it may be difficult in practicality. Asking for advice will be the next best option (B) as they may have experience with difficult patients. Asking the family for more information is an alternative option (E) which may give you a clue as to the nature of the patient's problems, but it is not the best option because it also mentions sending for an investigation that isn't always necessary. It would be wrong to treat the patient against their will (D) without first assessing their capacity, but worse to allow them home (C) without exploring what sinister causes could be affecting their cognition.

Question 67: ABDEC

We do not have enough information in the question to determine how important the blood results are, so we must assume they are important. Therefore, it would be best to call the team still at the hospital (A) so they can check them which may solve the problem quickly and directly. Failing this, unfortunately, patient safety must be your priority and you should return to check the bloods (B) since the results could warrant urgent treatment, and the delay of which could be very harmful to your patient. It is neutral to make a plan to ensure it does not happen again (D), because whilst this is a good thing to do, it does not solve the current situation. It is wrong to leave the bloods until the morning (E), but still worse to ignore them completely (C) as it is unlikely the results will be flagged up and so could be very damaging for the patient.

Question 68: EDCBA

In an ideal world, you would be able to leave at the end of your shift on time every day to ensure that you have enough rest between shifts, not only for your own benefit, but to ensure you are in a healthy state to make the best decisions for your patients. Although it is not a long-term solution, the best option in the case would be to stay (E) and complete jobs, as it is not clear whether (D) means the night FY1 will accept them. For a more long-term solution, the best option is to talk to your educational supervisors (C) who may be able to help you be more time-efficient during the day. The remaining two options are wrong because they do not deal with the current situation immediately, but of the two, (B) is worse than (A) as it achieves nothing except documenting to protect yourself.

Question 69: CABDE

The best option in this situation is to ask for help to safely complete the procedure (C). It deals with the current situation directly and finds a solution. The next best option is to explain (A) that you are not competent to perform it, although it does not find an immediate solution, it prevents you from doing something to a patient which you are not sure about, and may ensure the nurses contact another doctor to do the procedure. Refusing (B), whilst not immediately helpful to the patient, prevents you from causing them any further harm from performing an unknown procedure. Whilst doing your best to familiarise yourself before having a go (D) is better than trying without any more information (E) and documenting to protect yourself (E).

Question 70: ADF

In a social profession such as medicine, it is possible to understand how sometimes what could be first thought of as an attempt to socialise, could soon become drinking to excess in a slippery slope that is hard to notice. It is always best to discuss any concerns you have about your own health with your GP (D), as they can make an objective assessment of your drinking. It would also be prudent to ask your educational supervisor (F) at this stage, as although difficult to admit, they will then be in a better place to support you if they are aware of the situation. Taking a step back and reassessing the situation (A) to see where you can cut down drinking is a sensible step regardless of whether you have been drinking to excess or not. Asking your colleagues to stop making comments (B), or to apologise (H), does not attempt to address the issue here, which is your potential over drinking, whilst it may make you feel better. Discussing with a friend (E) is unhelpful as it is unlikely to yield an objective assessment. You should never attempt to treat or assess yourself (C), so this is inappropriate. Stopping drinking immediately (G) could seriously harm your health if indeed you are drinking, and in turn affect patients, so it is a very dangerous thing to do.

Question 71: BEDCA

Whilst it is very unlikely that the nurse is incorrect, it is still not okay for people who do not have permission to prescribe medicines and ask you to approve their decision later. The most important thing here is to ensure patient safety by checking the amount of fluid (B) and going to see the patient (E) to check on their status. Explaining that the nurse needs to ask for a prescription (D), will hopefully ensure such a situation does not arise again, but does not deal with the current risk immediately. The remaining answers are wrong as it is not just doctors that can sign prescriptions (C), but it would be the worst thing to do, in this case, to just sign the prescription (A) as it does not attempt to rectify the current or future situation. Whilst in some circumstances you may ask a nurse verbally for medication and sign for it retrospectively, there is no evidence that you have done so in this case.

Question 72: EDBAC

When providing medical information for patient's workplaces and insurance companies, it is important to balance the need for confidentiality with your honesty. In this situation, you should follow the GMC guidance that you should not leave out any "relevant information". It would be best to try and follow the guidance, which is to offer the patient the report (E) so they can decide whether to submit it to the company, because you cannot do so without their permission. Asking for a second opinion (D) in cases such as these where there is a dispute regarding information, the second doctor is almost certainly going to agree with your assessment on such objective information and may persuade the patient to realise that their request is unreasonable. It would be wrong to send a document with incorrect information, (B), but refusing to help without any sort of attempted compromise is unhelpful and may damage your relationship with the patient. Refusing to help the patient (A) because they are threatening you is denying the patient care but is better than sending the report (C) without their permission as it constitutes breaching confidentiality.

Question 73: EDBAC

In this scenario, it is important to handle the situation carefully. You have caught your colleague doing something he could likely be severely disciplined for, so it is best to confront the situation (E) and explain that you will escalate it if he does it again, which is likely to prevent him from doing so. Discussing the incident with the team (D) will likely ensure a quick resolution and protect the FY1 in question from severe punishment for what is hopefully an isolated incident. Escalating to the GMC (B) may mean that the situation is prematurely acted upon as the GMC will have to act as an authority to take some action and this is subordinate to talking to your colleague first. The remaining options essentially ignore the situation, but it is better to give the FY1 the benefit of the doubt (A) rather than becoming complicit and essentially asking them to bribe you for your silence (C).

Question 74: DCABE

The best option in this scenario is to check the medication from yesterday to ascertain whether you did indeed actually give the expired medicine (D) as you may be mistaken, which will prevent premature escalation of the incident without before ascertaining the facts. Raising the incident with the ward manager (C) will allow them to check the remaining stock and hopefully encourage them to realise that you were performing a task out of your normal duties. They may then put measures in place to prevent it happening again. It is important to be open about any mistakes and inform patients of them, so (A) is better than (B), because an incident form should be completed. The worst thing would be to not tell the patient (E), as they will not read their own medical notes so you would not be acting with candour, as is expected of you.

Question 75: EABCD

This is a difficult situation and is different to other issues of confidentiality because the threat posed to the wife is specific and grave enough to warrant breaking confidentiality if necessary. The best option is to encourage the patient to disclose the information (E). Asking for help is also a good option (A), but you should know the rules on disclosing a HIV status sufficiently to act yourself by this stage, but they may be able to help you to persuade the patient. It is true that you will be morally obliged to tell the patient's wife (B), but it would be far better for the patient to tell her himself. Telling the patient that you are going to break confidentiality (C) is a necessary step but it is less appropriate as it does not appear to offer the patient the opportunity to disclose the information himself. You cannot ignore this situation (D) as the risks involved are sufficient that not ensuring the information is disclosed would be negligent.

Question 76: DEF

There will often be stressful times when you are a doctor, and it is hard to manage your own feelings due to the levels of work. The best things to do when this happens are to take a short break to help you calm down (D), take a step back and reassess the tasks you have to complete (E), as well as thinking about what led to you becoming angry. Asking for help is always a good idea (F) as you are working as part of a team and your colleagues should offer to help if they can. In this situation, you should act as early as possible to prevent you becoming more frustrated to the extent where your work starts to suffer. Deferring responsibility to the nurses (A), medical students (H), or refusing to speak to family members is not appropriate (B). Whilst apologising to the family is a good idea (G), you should not do this so they don't complain, your motives should be more to rectify the situation. Leaving work could compromise patient care significantly (C) and this is not a serious enough situation to warrant this.

Question 77: EDCBA

The most important thing to do in this scenario is to protect the patient's safety. It is most appropriate to contact the consultant directly to check if this was a prescription error (E), as it may well have been on purpose. But secondary to this, until you are sure it was not a prescription error, you should change the prescription (D) to protect the patient from potential harm. At least this way you will be giving them potentially too little medicine rather than too much which is probably riskier. Leaving the dose as it is (C) potentially exposes the patient to an overdose of medication, but does also include the plan to check the dose to see if it is indeed an error. The remaining options are the wrong things to do, although it is mildly better to ask the nurses (B) about any other errors rather than cause the patient distress (A) without first checking all of the details.

Question 78: DECBA

Exploring the reasons behind the patient's sudden refusal (D) may reveal a simple fear that can be allayed. The next best thing is to inform your seniors (E) as they may be able to move onto another patient and prevent delays to the morning list. Moving the patient down the list (C) may give you more time to discuss the surgery with the patient, but is subordinate to the first two options. Cancelling the surgery (B) without exploring the patient's concerns is the wrong thing to do, but is better than coercing them into an operation (A), as you must respect the patient's right to refuse at any point, no matter how late on it is.

Question 79: DACBE

Completing death certificates are likely to form a common part of your role as a junior doctor. It is important to do so to the best of your ability and as honestly as possible. To just do as your consultant tells you would be the worst thing to do (E) if you do not agree. The best thing would be to discuss with your registrar (D) as they will almost certainly be able to offer helpful advice. This is because they may have known the patient better than the consultant and/or be able to help you if you then decide to go against the consultant's advice. Calling the coroner's office (A) is a good idea as they are always available to offer advice for these exact situations, but this is subordinate to asking your registrar first. Completing the form to the best of your knowledge (C) is the most honest thing to do but may harm your relationship with the consultant. Refusing to complete the certificate is the wrong thing to do (B) but is better than potentially writing down the wrong cause (E) as this is dishonest.

Question 80: BCEAD

This is a very difficult situation to handle. When you are the on-call doctor, you will often have to see new patients about whom you know very little. Deciding to give early supportive palliative care is increasingly being introduced, but the decision to remove treatment should be made considering the patient's, their family, and a multi-disciplinary approach. Coming in at this late stage may make you feel like you do not want to interfere with their treatment, but it is important not to prolong a patient's suffering that may have arisen due to a change in their condition. Hence the best thing to do is familiarise yourself with the case as much as possible (B). It may well be that a plan about fluids has been documented. The next best option would be to ask for advice from another doctor (C) as they may have more experience with such situations, but it is important that you understand the case before you do this, so it is less appropriate than (B). The remaining answers are all probably the wrong courses of action, explaining why the patient needs the fluids (E) may make the family agree to them through fear rather than it being in their best interests. Insisting on anything (A) is always the wrong thing to do but it is just better than stopping all of their medicines (D), which may cause the patient more harm and cause them to suffer.

Question 81: AEDBC

It is always best in these hard situations to try and find out more information (A). Asking for more information may give you a better idea and help you to decide how plausible their explanation may be. Contacting seniors (E) is very important as you will need their help with these situations and are unlikely to have sufficient experience to handle it alone, but it is important to establish more of the history before doing so. Contacting social services (D) is the next best option as they often have access to more information such as children being seen at other hospitals, but this should be done after the other two options. Confronting the mother (B) is less than ideal but better than delaying and not addressing the situation (A) as this could expose the child to more abuse in the meantime, which could have devastating consequences.

Question 82: ABCDE

In the increasing era of patients having access to the information about new medicines, it will become part of your role to explain the valid evidence about their status and why they are not being provided in certain cases. Here, the best option is to explore the patient's concerns (A) and be honest about the situation as this is likely to help them understand they have not been denied the drug. The next option (B) is subordinate to this because it does not explore the patient's concerns. Telling him to carry on (C) is neutral as it is not technically wrong, but does it not address their concerns. The remaining options are inappropriate as they are imparting false information that the drugs may help him (D) but this is better than saying they are too expensive (E) which would most likely make him very angry and damage your working relationship.

Question 83: AEDBC

Frequent attendees are difficult patients. Whilst it is hard to take them seriously as their number of attendances increases, it is important to not become blinded by their back story and ensure they are properly assessed every visit; they may well have chronic issues that recur often. The best approach is to ask for senior advice (A) as they will have experience of drug-seeking behaviour and be able to offer advice. As the patient is complaining of pain, you should give them the benefit of the doubt and prescribe analgesia (E). Reviewing later (D) is a neutral response as it may leave the patient in pain, but only temporarily and may give the previous dose of paracetamol time to kick in. Refusing pain relief as a junior is the wrong thing to do (B) but it is marginally better than reporting the patient (C) for what may turn out to be a chronic pain condition. It is important to try and give patients the benefit of the doubt as much as possible.

Question 84: CBDAE

The best thing to do when a confused patient is refusing an important investigation is to do a quick capacity assessment (C), as it may appear that the patient is perfectly competent for this decision. Explaining the risks (B) is the next best option because it could be that the patient is unsure why they are having the investigation and providing more information will help them understand. If in doubt, it is best to respect a patient's wishes (D) rather than subject them to investigations to which they are refusing, so this option places above the remaining two. Of the two worst options, it would be best to obtain the family of the patient's consent (A) rather than simply just disregarding their wishes (E).

Question 85: BCDEA

It is very important to give and receive a good handover at the start and end of shifts, as missed information could be very costly to your time and could compromise patient care. It is also important that you leave your shifts on time. In this case, the best option would be to answer and assess the request (B), as it may be a quick task that you can complete before the end of the shift, or if not, you will have the information to handover. Whilst it is noble to try and complete the task whatever the situation (C), it could be very time-consuming so it would be better to assess it. Asking the person bleeping (D) is a neutral response, as one would hope that if the task is sufficiently urgent, they would insist on you answering now. However, it delays the task by what may be crucial time. It would be wrong to ignore the bleep as it may be urgent, but it is better to mention it in your handover (E) than to ignore it completely (A), and answer it after, as it will impact on your work/life balance by delaying you more.

Question 86: ABDEC

Not only in a resource-limited NHS is it important to be thoughtful about investigations, but also to balance the need to allay patient's fears with the need to protect them from unnecessary investigations, especially those involving radiation. Asking for more information about the symptoms (A) may reveal the cause of the patient's concerns, or equally reveal information that would warrant the scan. That is why it is the best thing to do. Failing this, it would be best to explore the patient's ideas and concerns (B) as they may have a specific fear about which you can reassure. It is good to explain the risks of the scans (D) because patients are often not aware of these, but also to document that you have done this (E). However, this does not attempt to address her concerns so it is less than the ideal response. Equally, option (E) does not attempt to allay the concerns and the worst option would be to ignore these altogether (C) as their pain is not the primary concern at the moment.

Question 87: CDE

In this difficult situation, it is important to ensure that you take the patient's concerns very seriously and explain the complaints procedure (D) and that how lodging one does not affect her treatment. Asking for senior advice (E) is also a good idea as they will be able to help you to manage the situation sensitively and ensure you give the correct information. Escalating to the ward manager (C) is less than ideal at this stage as you are not sure there has been any wrongdoing, but is better than the incorrect remaining options. Offering to deal with the nurse yourself (A) (G) (F) is completely inappropriate as it would not be your place to discipline the nurse. Asking the patient to not make the complaint (B) is very unprofessional since it does not attempt to allay the patient's concerns nor make any attempt to prevent any potential recurrence. Telling the ward sister (H) would be appropriate, but not taking the matter further such as completing an incident form is the wrong thing to do.

Question 88: DACEB

Whilst it is important for you to teach, as it is how doctors learn much of their knowledge, it will often be difficult to do so and balance your patient's care. It is best to relay the concerns onto the department consultant as they will be responsible for the student's teaching programme (D). Failing this, you could offer to teach them (A) but this is not as good as going to the consultant as there may be a teaching programme available. Asking them to shadow another doctor (C) is a neutral response, because whilst it may help the students, it may put an unfair strain on your colleagues. Experiencing the wards is an invaluable part of the training, but in this instance, insisting on this (E) fails to address their concerns. Although, it is still better than giving them time off (B) as this may be against their medical school guidelines and could cause you problems if they escalate their concerns.

Question 89: CABDE

You may encounter patients who you believe to be making unwise medical decisions; this can range from doing harmful things such as excessively drinking and smoking to refusing medical treatment. It is not your job to lecture these patients but to explain the choices they are making as clearly as possible. Attending the current problem (C) is the main priority here. After this, it would then be best to explore the mother's concerns (A), as they may well have misconceptions about vaccinations that you could attempt to dispel. Explaining the benefits and risks of vaccinations (B) is also a good option, but does not make any mention of exploring the mother's current understanding. It is wrong to tell the mother that (D) the lack of vaccination has led to the condition because even if this is true, it is unlikely to help in any way, but it is better than refusing treatment (E), which is completely unacceptable and unprofessional.

Question 90: CDABE

This is a very precarious situation. Luckily, it appears that the patient has not had an anaphylaxis reaction but it is very important to stop the drug immediately (C) to prevent any further risk of harm. It would then be best to assess the patient to look for any signs of harm (D). Informing the ward sister will allow the process (A) to elucidate the errors in the process that allowed the error to happen. Completing the incident form (B) will be necessary as a patient has potentially been exposed to a lot of harm, however, this does not deal with the current situation. It would be completely inappropriate for you to tell off a nurse in this situation (E). If they are found to be at fault, there will be a disciplinary action scheme in place to deal with the matter, and it would be unprofessional for you to become involved.

Question 91: CADBE

Whilst not always practical, the guidance states that you should always have external translation for patients when you do not speak their language. It is often not a problem practically to allow patient's families to translate until you worry that the patient is not being fully informed about their care. In this case, the best option is to arrange for another appointment with an interpreter (C), where you can be sure the information will be communicated properly, especially with important news. The son may not have realised that he needs to translate precisely, and reminding him may prompt him to do so (A) is better than trying to ask the patient (D), as they are unlikely to say no, even if they understand you in the presence of their family. Whilst asking a member of staff who speaks their language would be a good thing to do, the issue here is that they do not speak the exact same language (B), and so the message may be lost. Continuing without an interpreter is likely to damage your relationship with the patient and their son, and it is the worst option as you are unlikely to be able to communicate the message effectively (E).

Question 92: BCH

Whilst commenting on your appearance may be embarrassing; the nurse is perfectly reasonable and should comment on any clothing that conflicts with the hospital policy with regards to professional dress and that which is required for infection control. Rules about items such as jewellery (C) and being bare below the elbows are required to protect patients, so the best thing for you to do would be to check the guidelines and see if you are dressed appropriately and explain this to the nurse (H). It would be good to ask your colleagues about whether you are dressed appropriately (B), as they may know more about the clothing regulations and be able to give you helpful feedback. The nurse has not necessarily said anything unprofessional (A) at this point, and to implicate your consultant too (D) is also wrong as you should follow the guidelines irrelevant of whether others do. Being a good doctor is important, but being one does not mean you can subvert the rules (E) or provide excuses (G) as they are there to protect patients. It would be very unethical to refuse to see patients (F) just because you feel insulted.

Question 93: BAECD

Parents are understandably concerned about their children, so in situations such as these where they may be being over worried, it is important to not dismiss their concerns and the best thing to do is to explore them (B). The next best thing is to explain (A), but this not as good as exploring their concerns. Refusing to prescribe the antibiotics and safety netting (E) is ultimately the correct thing to do but it is neutral, as it does not attempt to address the mother's concerns. Asking about home life (C) should be undertaken where you suspect any problems that may be leading to the mother's worries and is better than simply refusing the antibiotics (D) without any further resolution.

Question 94: EDBAC

With increasing pressure to move patients out of beds, it is important not to allow the pressure from ward managers and even more senior doctors to allow you to discharge patients before they are ready. In this case, it would be best to discuss this with a senior doctor (D) as they may be able to quickly advise you that such a result is nothing to worry about and allow you to safely discharge the patient, thus dealing with the situation quickly. Keeping the patient in (D) will protect them but may keep them in unnecessarily. Nonetheless, it is a safe option but subordinate to trying to deal with it quickly. Discussing this with the patient is unhelpful (B) as they are unlikely to understand the intricacies of the blood result. This does however leave the potential option for the patient to be kept in as opposed to the remaining options. Discharging with a follow-up (A) should safeguard the patient from harm, from what appears to be a fairly minor electrolyte imbalance and is better than letting them go (C) without any sort of follow up.

Question 95: DEACB

Poor compliance with medications is a common problem you will encounter whether through ignorance or defiance. Assuming that this patient has capacity, which one must do with adults until proven otherwise, she is perfectly entitled to make medical decisions, regardless of whether you feel they are unwise. However, you should try to inform her about the consequences of the choices she is making (E), but this is secondary to treating her current problem (D), which are the best two options. Providing written information can be a useful tool (A), but does not give the patient the opportunity to ask questions, so should be used in addition to a face-to-face discussion. Not offering any further advice is the wrong thing to do (C), but is better than breaking her confidentiality and undermining her to her relatives which is the worst option.

Question 96: CGH

Whilst it is important to honour your academic commitments, it must not come at a compromise to patient care. In this scenario, it is important that you do not stay up so late that you become tired and are not at your best the next day (B) (D). It would be best to explain to your consultant (C) that you will do your best to finish tomorrow (H) and give them an accurate timeline for when you can finish (G). They should then be reasonable and give you some more time. Asking for help (A) is unfair as it is your work and will put extra work on your colleague unfairly. Staying up late and calling in sick (B) is a very inappropriate thing to do as it may leave your team understaffed. Asking your consultant to help you (E) is not the worst option, but passing the responsibility of finishing it is less appropriate than the correct answers. Lying to them about personal problems (F) is unprofessional.

Question 97: ACBDE

The best thing is to ask for reaffirmation from your colleagues (A). They may well have noticed the consultant's appearance today but might not feel like they can say anything. Approaching the consultant directly is the next best step (C), but it would be better to ask your colleagues first as you can then approach him as a team with your concerns, which would be harder to ignore. Asking for advice from other colleagues (B) is a neutral response as it is unlikely they will have the experience to handle the situation and does not immediately deal with the problem. Reporting the consultant (D) is an extreme step and should only be attempted when other, more direct actions have failed as you do not have any evidence that there is harm to patients at this stage. Ignoring the situation (E) is the worst thing to do as there may be harm to patients in the meantime.

Question 98: ACG
It is important to be honest with this patient, but that does not mean you should make them feel like they are not worthy of certain investigations (H). You should not lie and explain things that you do not understand (A). Being honest and explaining that you are not sure why they have been ordered a particular investigation (C) is the right thing to do, especially with the added promise to find out more information. Using this as a learning situation is also a good thing to do (G). Deferring explaining to the radiologists (B) (D), is unlikely to be successful and is not a fair use of their time. Whilst a patient cannot demand treatment when it is not medically indicated, telling them they cannot have a certain investigation without explanation (E) is not helpful. Making a note to ask about the scan the next day (F) does not solve the current problem.

Question 99: AEDBC
In this situation, it is always best to clarify what prompted the other person's statements (A). It may have simply been an offhand remark or a reflection of their stresses rather than a comment on your own. Seeking medical advice (E) is the next most appropriate step as it is better to get an objective assessment of your mental health. The next best thing to do would be to discuss this with your supervisor (D) as they can help you to be more time-efficient or help you with coping strategies. It is less than ideal to ask other FY1s for their opinions (B) as this may result in adding to your stress rather than allaying it, but it is better than attempting to self-medicate (C), as you should never attempt to treat yourself.

Question 100: EACDB
Patient safety is the primary responsibility in all cases such as this. Just because you do not believe patient safety is compromised, you may not have the experience to make that decision. Approaching the registrar directly (E) may allow you to gather more information as to the nature and cause of the behaviour. If that fails, asking a senior in confidence for advice on how to proceed (A) is a pragmatic option. Ultimately, the consultant who supervises the registrar is the next best option (C) and is better than discussing and speculating with your colleagues (D). Escalation to the GMC should be the last resort and usually beyond your remit except in extreme circumstances (B).

Question 101: BDCEA
Patient safety is of utmost priority even if they are irate (B). Then the most appropriate course is to apologise to them (D). Documentation should be done as soon as possible as this increases accuracy and detail of events (C). Giving the patient information on how to register a complaint (E), should then be completed before informing their respective consultant (A).

Question 102: DACBE
It is clearly stated by the GMC that one should avoid treating friends and family unless absolutely essential, and these are very common requests. This is clearly not a life-threatening scenario. (D) is the most appropriate response and offers a solution should he truly want the antibiotics. (A) is preferable to (C) because sending someone to A&E is an inappropriate use of resources, particularly as there is no apparent indication for the antibiotics. (B) is the next most appropriate response. The GMC states that, if you prescribe medications for someone close to you, you need to make a record at the time, which includes your relationship to the patient and why it was necessary for you to prescribe the medication. Then you are required to tell the patient's GP which medicines you have prescribed and any other necessary information. (E) is the worst as it is clearly theft.

Question 103: CBAED

This is a tough, but sometimes common scenario. As your education is being affected, talking to your educational supervisor would be best, and also has the advantage that they are outside of the team (C). Your clinical supervisor should be next as it involves a group of trainees so it will need to be approached from a higher level (B). Organising a meeting could be a constructive exercise but can be difficult when it involves multiple people (A). Normally, a foundation programme director is the last point of call and should only be involved after other avenues are exhausted (E). Sending a message on the messaging application is not ideal because it does not tackle the problem, could be interpreted badly, and could isolate you further, therefore, being the lowest (D).

Question 104: DEBCA

This is a very common scenario, and in most cases, it is professional to wait to give a direct verbal handover (D). However, handing over to another colleague on that shift is an alternative, but remember, they may not be responsible for those patients (E). Writing a list is always advisable and leaving it somewhere that is easily accessible is prudent (B). This is better than calling them later which may lead to you forgetting details and certain jobs that need to be handed over, particularly if there are time critical jobs (C). Emailing is pointless, especially as here it is not stated that they have been made aware of what you have done (A).

Question 105: ABCED

Prioritisation is a common facet of your working day. In this case, it is prudent to finish seeing the patient in A&E and complete all those tasks as you may forget later which can be a patient safety issue (A). Then you should ask the charge nurse in A&E as the drug chart may be to hand, which can then be sent to the ward (B). It also serves as a way of making the charge nurse aware of the potential lapse in care. Rewriting a drug chart ensures the patient is able to get analgesia, but because you are certain you have written one already, it can also become a safety issue if they receive too much medication (C). Filing an incident report should be next (E). Discussing with the matron does not have a direct impact on patient safety at this point but can be done, usually only after speaking to the nurses themselves (D).

Question 106: EDCBA

Thanking the patient is the first thing you should do before politely declining (E, D). Asking for a communal gift is preferable to making a donation purely based on your behalf as there are many people involved in patient care (C, B). Buying gifts yourself is a nice thought, but does involve you accepting the cash sum, making it the least preferable option (A).

Question 107: ABDCE

In this scenario, protecting the child is your primary concern. You should involve your supervisor at the earliest opportunity before taking a full history and performing a witnessed head to toe examination (A, B). Once this is done, completing full and accurate documentation with phrases, dates, and times is essential as this can be used in court (D). You should inform and obtain advice from the designated individual for child protection about how to proceed (C). As the partner is non-resident and not present at the consultation, informing the police is not an imminent priority until further advice is sought (E).

Question 108: BDCAE
In this case, patient and staff safety is paramount. Notifying the patient that they cannot smoke is usually sufficient, and offering an alternative, particularly for heavy smokers is a good compromise (B, D). Some patients can get aggressive so asking for assistance from security personnel is advisable (C). Confiscating his lighter is an extreme, usually temporising, measure but should be done to protect other patients (A). Letting him smoke is not acceptable (E).

Question 109: ABECD
Distressed families can potentially be very difficult to deal with. Attempting to de-escalate the situation by apologising and reasoning can sometimes be enough (A, B). If the family are still aggressive, it can be worth stepping back, informing security and asking another individual to speak to them (E, C, D).

Question 110: ABCDE
In this scenario, the critical care outreach nurse has no reason to be looking through the patient notes, especially as they are not involved in the patient's care. It is usually best to approach the person directly (A). It should also be escalated to the nurse in charge before submitting an incident report (B, C). The information governance team will need to be informed (D). This usually occurs after submitting an incident report. You should not submit a PALS complaint as this is a patient advice and liaison service (E).

Question 111: CEDAB
Inappropriate workplace behaviour is sadly commonplace. Approaching the person causing the problems can be useful as it could be easily resolved with a simple conversation (C). If this doesn't settle, then utilise your clinical supervisor and the rota coordinator (E, D). Putting up with the comments is never a good solution but using humour can diffuse tension rather than saying nothing (A, B).

Question 112: CEDBA
This is a suboptimal situation but is not that uncommon in practice as you become more senior. In this case, the two best options are first to contact the patient's family to notify them and see if you can find out whether a discussion has been held (C). Then, seeking the advice of the palliative care service is always valuable for advice on symptom control (E). In the absence of a plan, you should use an element of clinical judgement as resuscitation may not be in the patient's best interests (D). Filling in a DNAR should always be done by the most senior person available, but it is preferable in this case, particularly if you have spoken to the family, to stopping all the medications. This should not be an individual decision (B, A).

Question 113: BCDAE
Being offered multiple projects to do is a common scenario in medicine, particularly when it comes to audit. Being honest is the most acceptable. You should not place too much burden on yourself – and offering to find someone else is a reasonable answer because it proposes a solution for the consultant (B, C). Ideally, you should never be in a position to give up your free time to do the projects, so, therefore, not bringing up the subject again is better than agreeing (D, A). Doing this project at the expense of others makes you unreliable and untrustworthy (E).

Question 114: ABCED
This concerns when it is okay to breach confidentiality. As a medical professional, you should initially advise the patient of what they need to do when they have epilepsy (A, B). If the patient is not willing to contact the DVLA then you should inform them you will have to before doing so (C, E). You should not really involve the patient's partner without the patient's consent as this is a breach of confidentiality (D).

Question 115: CADEB
Again, you should approach the person in question if you feel comfortable doing so and give them the chance to apologise and own up to their misdemeanour (C). If not, then involving a trusted senior colleague is useful before escalating to the consultant (A, D). Doing nothing is preferable to blackmailing the individual (E, B).

Question 116: ACDEB
Your priority is the patient in this scenario and the most reasonable response would be to have a discussion with her in private (A). If you suspect domestic abuse – particularly if there is a physical element – then a full examination is warranted which should be documented as soon as is reasonably practicable (C, D). Asking her to book a follow-up delays potential exploration of the problem and could endanger her (E). Broaching the subject whilst the partner is there is not appropriate seeing as the patient left the room to notify your team (B).

Question 117: CDBAE
In order to assess the situation and treat in that patient's best interest, it may be necessary to perform a mental capacity assessment (C). The next best choice depend upon how unwell the patient is, but giving oral antibiotics could be lifesaving and less aggravating before attempting to physically restrict or sedate then cannulate (D, B, A). The final option is not really appropriate unless you deem that the patient does have capacity (E).

Question 118: AEDBC
Euthanasia is a current topic that is hotly debated. In the UK, Physician-assisted suicide is illegal. So, here you should explore why the patient feels like that and then see if there is any way you can treat his symptoms utilising available senior resources – up the chain before going across (A, E, D). The last two answers depend upon the clinical scenario. By utilising the doctrine of double effect, increasing his analgesia in a carefully titrated way is an acceptable response but doubling it is usually too great a change, making it the least appropriate choice here (B, C).

Question 119: BCDEA
Translation services can be variable. In this case, a gentle reminder to the translator may be sufficient (B), otherwise, the use of another translator may be required (C) - the procedure will not take place until the patient is adequately consented. (D) is the next most appropriate action. Rebooking the outpatient appointment is appropriate but may delay the procedure for a period of time and family members bring their own challenges when translating (E). Asking for signed consent is completely inappropriate (A).

Question 120: CBDAE
Drug-seeking behaviour is common and cyclizine is one the most commonly sought-after medications. It is important to establish why they are refusing other anti-emetics, for example, intolerance or no effect and what is better about cyclizine (C, B). If stuck, asking for advice on prescribing an alternative is wise (D). Using omeprazole as a placebo is deceitful (A, E).

Question 121: CDABE
Asking the patient should be your first point of call as there may be another reason for why he doesn't want to leave (C). Discharging with a point of contact is good for regular attendees and gives them a means of accessing help quickly in the community (D). Discharging the patient is better than not and involving the social services team as there is very little they can do (A, B). Asking your SHO to see the patient will not change a decision on whether to discharge or not, and will be of no benefit (E).

Question 122: BEDCA
Doctors are at a very high risk of developing alcohol dependency due to the nature of the job. In this case, patient safety is your main concern. You should give your colleague the opportunity to respond for his behaviour and take it upon himself to notify his seniors (B). If he doesn't act, patient safety is at risk and therefore it should be promptly escalated (E). Discussing it with peers is an intermediate step. However, it can result in unnecessary delays in reporting if you wait for a recurrence (D, C). The last option is an attempt to cover up their actions and, as such, indirectly condones it (A).

Question 123: CEDBA
As a junior, this is a common scenario as there will be diagnoses that you will not have come across. Being open and honest is essential and being proactive in trying to get the results so another can come and explain them is encouraged (C, E). Once you have the results available, a senior can then come and discuss them (D). Researching the investigations is beneficial to your learning for the future, but reading numbers to a patient will likely be unintelligible for the patient, thus, (B) is preferred to (A).

Question 124: DCEBA
In some cases such as these, there may be a logical explanation that you have not factored in, e.g. organ dysfunction, so asking is the best idea (D). Printing off the guidelines and asking the pharmacy is valuable if you want to double check and the consultant hasn't given you a clear answer (C, E). Changing the antibiotics later is dangerous without consulting someone (B), but so is not making a change if you think the prescription risks patient safety (A).

Question 125: ECDBA
As with any patient who may be deteriorating, you should do a proper assessment and instigate potentially lifesaving treatments, then conduct investigations to aid your diagnosis (E, C, D). If your registrar is busy, trying to get advice from the medical team is a good idea and critical care outreach can be used as a backup should they be required/ anaesthetic input warranted (B, A).

Question 126: CABED
Documenting your conversation in the notes is an accurate representation of events, whereas speaking to the patient then documenting gives the impression you had consent and could be seen as being deceitful. Therefore, (A) is preferable to (B). (C) is clearly the best route to take regardless. Not documenting anything leaves you liable to litigation but is better than outright falsification that you had the patient's consent (E, D).

Question 127: ECDBA
Option (E) is ideal as this is an emergency and you are contributing to patient care in a safe way. (C) is an alternative because you are helping with patient workload but not the patient most at risk. (D) is true but doesn't offer a solution. (B) is a safer option than (A) as you should never be the only person consenting the patient. It is less desirable than the others as you should avoid being put in a position to consent if at all possible.

Question 128: ADBEC
Approaching your colleague directly is usually the best option (A) if done in a sympathetic manner, but failing this, a direct senior is a good alternative option (D). If this doesn't work, discussing it with the consultant in charge of your team would be the next level if not resolved (B). Educational supervisors are not usually involved in clinical matters as this falls under the clinical supervisor remit (C). And although camaraderie is encouraged in the profession, it is not a requirement, meaning (E) is better than (C), although not for you in this case.

Question 129: ACBDE
The obvious first step is to notify security and then try to talk the patient down and de-escalate the situation (A, C). If that fails, then the safety of other patients is a concern and they should be moved out of the way of harm (B). Sedating the patient should only be used as a last resort due to associated risks (D). You should not attempt to restrain a patient without appropriate training (E).

Question 130: EBDAC
Likely to become more common in the future. Sending a message that extends thanks is more suitable than just sending a letter saying why you could not add them (E, B). The GMC clearly states that you should avoid engaging patients on social media, so not adding them at all is an appropriate response and you, as a junior doctor, will be expected to have this knowledge (D). Adding them is the worst of the answers, certainly worse than consulting your colleagues (A, C).

Question 131: CEBAD
Information governance is an important concept and one that commonly occurs. In this case, you simply may have misplaced the list within the hospital so asking your colleagues if they have seen it could locate it (C). If not, you should notify your consultant that there is a potential loss of confidential information and then submit an incident report (E, B). Printing off a new list is better than stealing another colleague's (A, D).

Question 132: ACDEB
Apologising to the patient should always be your first port of call, making sure that you do not use language that puts the weight of the mistake upon yourself (A). Then you should inform your registrar and ask them to come and review the patient (C, D). An incident report should be submitted, but this can happen further down the line (E). You shouldn't be put in the position of breaking the bad news to the patient, particularly if they are already upset.

Question 133: EABCD
This question tests the concept of capacity and right of a patient to choose what happens to them. Remember that you must be unbiased in your judgement and by empathising with both sides, this will create trust between the two (E). Then you should highlight that every patient has the right to choose what happens to them although you try to take family wishes into account when possible (A, B). Clearly documenting the full conversation is important, including the benefits and drawbacks that you have covered (C). You should never assume that a patient does not have capacity unless you perform an official assessment (D).

Question 134: DCEBA
In this scenario, the registrar is performing an illegal activity which is worse considering they are supposed to be responsible for child welfare. You should inform the site practitioners immediately (D) and then the on call consultant (D). The GMC should be informed after raising concerns with your manager or an appropriate officer and you are not satisfied that the responsible person has taken adequate action (E). A GMC investigation is likely to be protracted so it is better to do (D) and (C) as they will result in more rapid action. You should avoid confronting the registrar directly (B) – this is unlikely to resolve the issue and will likely put you in a difficult position. Feigning ignorance is not an acceptable response (A) given the risk of long term harm arising.

Question 135: BCADE
It goes without saying in this case that you should begin aggressive fluid resuscitation first (B). Asking what the child would like is valuable as they are your patient, however, they may not be in a physiological state to have capacity and at that age, a parent is usually always required for consent unless Gillick competent (C). In life-threatening scenarios, however, despite parental wishes, your priority is the child and you should always act in their best interests (A). Contacting the legal team should be done at a later stage (D). Not giving the patient blood could endanger their life (E).

Question 136: ABDEC
All patients with depression should be screened for suicidal ideation regardless of the history, this should then be discussed with you senior (A, B). She is a patient at risk and so an urgent psychiatric assessment is needed to see whether she needs to be admitted or sectioned under the mental health act for treatment (D). Starting her on antidepressant medication will not be immediate as it will only help over a period of 6 weeks, and a referral to social services will also take time (E, C).

Question 137: BCDAE
In this case, the correct order depends on whether you feel the patient is Gillick competent. To judge this, you must establish capacity – the ability to understand, retain, weigh up and repeat the information you provide (B, C, D). Whether you prescribe the medication or not is fully dependent on this. Although you feel she is, you must go through the stages of assessment first rather than assuming she is (A). Involvement of the mother is only necessary if she does not have capacity to make that decision (E).

Question 138: ABCED
Immediately in cases such as these, resuscitation should be started aggressively with prompt senior input (A, B). Contacting the next of kin is only useful in life or death scenarios and their feelings shouldn't alter your initial clinical management (C). You should avoid filling in a DNACPR, but more so palliating patients without at least discussing with your seniors (E, D).

Question 139: EABDC

Regardless of whether a patient is private, if you are there and they are unstable you should always review them (E). If you are not happy to do so, then asking them to call the SHO is a reasonable alternative (A). Medico-legal and asking for compensation should come later (B, D). Declining to see a sick patient is not acceptable (C).

Question 140: DCAEB

If a patient has been listed for an inpatient colonoscopy, the best thing is to see if it can be expedited, at least then you can update the patient and let them make a more informed decision (D). If the patient wants to go privately, normally a consultant will make the appropriate arrangements and you shouldn't have to (C). If you are struggling, ask a clinical supervisor for advice as they could point you in the right direction (A). For the last two options, (E) is more proactive than (B).

Question 141: EDBCA

This is a typical breaking bad news situation. Explaining the rationale is the best way to start, followed by breaking the news (E, D). There would normally be a pause for questions before detailing a preliminary plan (B). A detailed sexual history is important but using it as an opening gambit would be awkward, especially as you have the test results (C). Referring for further treatment in this case is the last priority (A).

Question 142: DCBAE

This relates to the principle of breaking confidentiality for the 'greater good of the public'. The surgical registrar has the responsibility to tell the occupational health department, if not, you should notify them (D, C). The next option is to notify their supervising consultant, then regional director, then GMC (B, A, E).

Question 143: CEABD

This question is related to patient confidentiality. Before discussing anything, the patient should be consented (C). If the results haven't been given to the patient, you cannot give them to the family but you can say if they are ready for discharge (E, A). Taking responsibility to break the bad news is better than passing the phone on (B, D).

Question 144: CDEAB

In this case, you are the more senior person on the take. Although it is not appropriate, you are without registrar support, therefore, the site managers/practitioners should be notified early (C). You should speak to your colleague and say that they do not have the experience to act up (D, E). As an intermediate measure, you should carry the bleep but this is suboptimal (A). The last option does not solve any problems, but may create them (B).

Question 145: CBEAD

In this case, not an uncommon one, your clinical supervisor is key in ensuring the even distribution of workload across the team (C). The next best option is the registrars, although their decisions carry less weight (B). Then you could ask for your educational supervisor's input as this is impacting on your learning opportunities and career development (E). Sending an angry message to the group will not provide a solution and may create further problems (A). However, (D) is the worst response and goes against GMC guidance, which states that we must treat colleagues fairly and with respect. The standards expected of doctors do not change because they are communicating through social media rather than face to face and (D) would certainly damage the public's trust in the profession.

Question 146: BCADE
None of these answers are the optimal way of dealing with the issue. Helping out the other team is a good place to start but doesn't fix the problem of the job. Therefore, contacting the foundation programme director to review the post is wise (B, C). Performing quality improvement has the potential to be better for patients than studying for an exam, making it a better option (A, D). Spending the time in the mess is not a good option (E).

Question 147: EDACB
Irate and aggressive patients are a common clinical occurrence. In this case, as the nurse has come to you about it, you should speak to the patient directly and ask them to apologise if practicable (E, D). They should also escalate to the matron (A). Changing bays is an option and better than the other as it still ensures the patient receives clinical care (C, B).

Question 148: DCBEA
In patients who are challenging and threaten litigation, documentation is crucial (D). Ideally, you should see the patient in groups although this is not the best answer as it is not always practicable in reality (C). Before considering an operation, legal input would be wise (B). The last two options are both suboptimal. However, not seeing the patient on a ward round will do less harm than the patient having an operation which is not clinically indicated (E, A).

Question 149: ABCDE
This question relates to confidentiality and protecting the "public's interest." Initially, you should put the onus on the patient to have to deliver the information (A). Telling the patient that you need to advise their partner at least gives them the opportunity to have the conversation themselves, and informs them that you will be breaching their confidentiality should you need to (B). Arranging a mutual appointment may allow the conversation to happen in a supported environment (C). Use of barrier contraception is a later step to prevent further transmission and does not directly relate to the principle of the question (D). However, the last answer is clearly inappropriate (E).

Question 150: CEADB
The GMC clearly states that you should avoid treating friends and relatives if at all possible. The most appropriate response is to ask her to see her GP followed by refusing to give advice (C, E). Sending her to A&E is an inappropriate use of resources and if she did go, you shouldn't be seeing her there (A). You are an FY1 and cannot write a private prescription, but this is better than advising theft (D, B).

Question 151: DBCAE
This is a straightforward case whereby prescriptions are dependent on the blood results. Start by explaining to the nursing staff you cannot do it without the INR result, then chase the result in the lab (D, B). If it is not back by the end of your shift then you should hand the job over (C). Dosing the same as the day before is risky but ignoring the request is a worse answer (A, E).

Question 152: DCBEA
If a patient has capacity then they are able to refuse consent including to cannulation, therefore, asking another person to do it is appropriate (D, C). In this case, the patient has a valid reason to refuse, so a capacity assessment would not necessarily be required (B). Walking away is the worst option as the patient needs antibiotics and you will not remedy that by just documenting this in your notes (E).

Question 153: BFH

(B) is the most compassionate response and allows you to explore the problem. If she is having trouble at home, her GP is the best source of support (H). Ultimately, if her training is being affected, she should involve her educational supervisor (F). In this case, it is not appropriate for you to judge whether she is fit for work or should take sick leave.

Question 154: DEF

(D) is the natural response to such an incident. The paediatric team will be experienced in dealing with teenagers in this scenario (E). Remember, Gillick competence only relates to consenting to treatment, it does not allow children to refuse it. (F) is a reasonable tactic that can be employed fairly quickly and effortlessly (assuming his friends are reasonable). Any answers relating to discharge are unsafe. Calling his parents without informing him is breaching his confidentiality, so is less optimal than the other available options. In practice, if you were to call his parents you should inform him you are doing so.

Question 155: ABD

(A) is naturally what your first response would be. Exploring ideas, concerns, and expectations is an important process when developing management plans (B). In this case, the child is old enough to be involved in the decision to commence treatment and it would be useful to gain their insight into whether/how the condition is affecting them (D). It would be important to explain the advantages and disadvantages of treatment, but only if you decide the treatment is warranted, which in this case it is unlikely to be.

Question 156: BDE

An urgent psychiatric assessment would be required in order to determine whether this patient needs to be treated under the mental health act (D) and (B) follows on from the this. Seniors would likely have more experience in managing cases such as this, which are more common than you may believe, therefore asking for senior review (E) is also an appropriate option. Asking for medico-legal advice is prudent but should not delay your assessment and decision to start treatment. Respecting her rights or discharging is not appropriate as the patient has suicidal ideation. This would not come under the mental capacity act unless the patient was acutely confused, e.g. with encephalopathy or intoxication.

Question 157: ACH

First and foremost, you must ensure the patient is fully informed before they can make the decision to refuse treatment (H). Regardless of whether or not you will transfuse, (A) should be done so it is available. In this case, there isn't time to take a more calculated legal approach as they are in extremis. You should therefore treat in the best interests (C) followed by a mental capacity assessment afterwards. Auto transfusion is not appropriate if there is a catastrophic haemorrhage. Calling the relatives can be useful but not in an emergency scenario like this.

Question 158: BDE

If a patient has appendicitis then, as the FY2, you would be expected to explain the condition and why they need the procedure (D). Naturally, the registrar should consent the patient if you are unable to (E). Refusing to consent the patient is an acceptable response (B). You should not try to explain a procedure if you do not understand the complications and risks.

Question 159: BDG

(B) is the most appropriate response and will allow you to gain insight into their perspective. Obviously, workload is shared among the team and so you should seek and value their opinion (D). (G) is a proactive way of showing that you have taken on board their constructive criticism. The fact that this is your first job is an acceptable answer to an extent, but does not show a willingness to improve, therefore, is not one of the top three. There is no evidence that this is a sign of bullying. As this relates to clinical work, your educational supervisor would not be the right person to involve.

Question 160: BDE

Gaining their side of the story is valuable before attempting to escalate or have a group discussion as they may feel this behaviour is affecting patient safety (D). (B) is the best solution to the problem as this is clearly a professionalism issue that could be resolved among the team. The clinical supervisor is ultimately responsible for harmony within the team and if there is a disjointed relationship, they need to know and address the issue (E). Changing teams is one option but will not solve the problem between the two people on the small team. The medical education department would not get involved until later, nor would the foundation programme director.

Question 161: CGH

An obvious case may be that the item has been misplaced and is easily retrievable. Therefore (C) should be done before accusing or searching through other patient's belongings. (H) is the best option as the item may have been found and locked away for safe keeping. Sending an email to all the ward staff may again identify someone who has found the item and put it away for safe keeping (G). Dismissing the case is inappropriate even if the patient does have dementia. Involving security and the police would only be done after a thorough search does not reveal anything. Submitting a PALS complaint would be appropriate if nothing is found.

Question 162: DFG

(D) is the most important first step in gathering information. If the midwives are unhappy, the head midwife is their port of call and they should be involved either via the midwives or yourself (F). The matron has more control over the nursing and doctor personnel, so would be a good intermediary between the doctor's side and the midwives (G). In this case, it would not be your responsibility to speak to the consultant directly or apologise on their behalf. Involving your clinical supervisor could be an alternative to speaking to the matron of obstetrics and gynaecology.

Question 163: BEF

This is a difficult case as there is potential for impact on patient safety and experience. If you can, the best would be to find a solution with your registrar (E). If this fails, then asking for colleague input would be important (F). Escalating to the consultant would come after asking for colleague input (B). Moving rotations would be a radical step. Again, this is not impacting the education side of training so notifying the educational supervisor is not warranted at this stage.

Question 164: DEG

In this case, you should make it evident that the language the core trainee used was inappropriate (D). Notifying the ward sister is also prudent as it allows them to be aware should any complaint be put in (E). Ultimately, you should inform your consultant who could then decide if action is needed (G).

Question 165: BCD

Note that this question asks for the least appropriate options. (B) will not achieve anything. (C) is also inappropriate as you should not attempt to blackmail the person involved. In addition, as there is no evidence of alcohol dependency, emailing occupational health would not be appropriate (D). All the other options are valid, although (F) and (G) should be later down the chain of escalation.

Question 166: ABF

This question relates to being open and honest but also not risking patient safety – in the case of tiredness. (B) is the most sensible option, whilst (F) is also sensible. (C) is the most appropriate third answer, as (G) is lying and (D, E) risk patient safety. (C) is thoughtful but does not address the issue of you being late or apologising.

Question 167: CGH

This is fairly common when asked or told to do tasks that are menial and no one else more senior wants to take responsibility for them. (G) is the most appropriate as it may galvanise them to do their share so they are not embarrassed. (H) is another appropriate way of dividing labour so that you are not over-burdened unfairly. (C) is a better option than (F) as you should not be in a position to do this on your own.

Question 168: BFG

This is a scenario where it may be best to avoid approaching the person directly without substantial evidence, as stealing a controlled drug is theft and may be a sign of opiate addiction, which could put their career in jeopardy. The most appropriate action is to escalate this if you have any suspicions and allow others to investigate it (G, B). Gathering evidence from other trainees may support your suspicion/allegation (F). Notifying the pharmacist is also a pragmatic approach to initiating an investigation, but doesn't deal with the fact that you are suspicious about a certain doctor.

Question 169: CFH

By doing some reading and improving your own learning, you may be able to provide a good teaching session for the medical students, making (H) the best option. Appreciably, this is not always practicable so changing the topic is a valid response (C). (F) would also be an acceptable response and superior to (A) as it gives a method by which the students get teaching rather than having it cancelled. Rearranging the teaching should only occur if nobody is free to do it.

Question 170: ADE

In this case, there may be reasons for ordering the investigations about which you are not aware of, therefore, getting the consultant's input is advisable (A). If you are finding this a regular problem, then approaching your clinical supervisor, who is usually within the same specialty, may allow this to be discussed at a higher level (E). Ultimately, patients should choose what investigations to have, so it would also be reasonable to ask their opinions providing that you give them all the options and full explanations of the risks and benefits (D). If you suspect patient safety is at risk, you have a duty to whistle blow in some way, meaning (G) is not appropriate. (C) may cause harm if you do not know the indications fully and (H) is not practicable in the NHS.

Question 171: CDG
In this case, your clinical supervisor and educational supervisors should both be involved as it is affecting your progression and experience (D, C). (G) is preferable to (B) as it means you are staying within your specialty and being proactive about obtaining better experiences. Reflecting would be useful later on when you have attempted to make a change. (H) is a lazy option.

Question 172: ABD
In this case, all team members have a responsibility to reduce transmission of hospital-acquired pathogens (D). Making sure your personal practice is up to standard is the first step, but deficiencies by multiple people means it needs to be raised at a higher level – the most appropriate being the director of the department (B). Listing the findings for discussion is a proactive way for the department to respond and seek improvement (A). (E) is not an ideal answer as it involves many people and puts the onus on you to be responsible for everyone's practice, which is not sustainable in the long run.

Question 173: ABF
Asking the consultant why they think your dress is inappropriate is the first way to proceed, so long as the conversation is had in a professional manner (B). You should also ask your colleagues about what they feel regarding your dress as it may only be one member who feels you dress inappropriately (F). (A) will support you on how to proceed. Changing and shopping is excessive unless this is repeatedly mentioned by several different team members.

Question 174: BDG
This is affecting your educational experience so you should raise it with your educational supervisor (D). As the rota problem is within the department, you should also speak to your clinical supervisor (G). Patient safety may be at risk, but this is not going to be resolved by you covering the shifts all the time due to the effects of fatigue. Therefore, (B) is an appropriate response until people are appointed to the post.

Question 175: ADECB
The safety of the patient is paramount and if you have arranged a blood transfusion, there must be a good clinical indication for it – particularly for it to happen overnight! Therefore, you should try to contact the FY1 who would be responsible for it first, and if not, the nursing staff looking after the patient as they can arrange it as well (A, D). Your next port of call would be the on call registrar (E). (B) is the worst option as the blood would not last overnight, leaving going in yourself as the second worst (C).

Question 176: DEBAC
In cases of antibiotic prescribing, most trusts have robust guidelines on their intranet (D). If these are not available out of hours, you could ask your registrar and if they do not know, you should contact the microbiology consultant (E, B). The out of hours pharmacist does not usually have a role in deciding the antibiotics prescribed but can give advice on what organisms can be covered by certain drugs (A). They may also know the protocol depending on their area of specialty. The BNF has a section on generic antibiotics that you can use in certain infections, but this should not be relied upon as it can significantly differ from your trust protocols (C).

Question 177: DCEBA

In this case, again, patient safety is the main priority. The best thing to do would be to hand over the jobs and leave (D) followed by informing the registrar to whom you are responsible that you are going (C). The next best option would be to complete the urgent jobs then leave (E). Of the last two, taking an anti-emetic is preferable as although it is stealing, it will allow some symptomatic relief for yourself (B, A). However, both options are bad.

Question 178: CEBDA

In this case, when an advanced directive exists and you are unable to fully communicate with a patient, you should not, nor should you be responsible for, filling in a DNAR form (C). You should attempt to arrange the transfer of the DNAR form before seeking advice from your legal department regarding the contents and how to proceed (E, B). If a DNAR is to be completed, it should be signed by the most senior person and by a consultant within 24 hours (D). As stated, you should not fill one yourself (A).

Question 179: ADCEB

This is a patient safety issue and you have made the medication changes based on an appropriate clinical context. You should engage the nursing staff to see if they have a reason to be giving the old doses (A). If there isn't a valid clinical reason, you should escalate it to the nurse in charge or ward sister and fully document the conversations you have had in the notes (D, C). In this case, the error is not your fault so apologising is lower down. The nursing staff should be the ones to apologise, but from a professional perspective, it is still courteous (E). Finally, you should complete an incident report (B).

Question 180: CBADE

As you need the meeting in order to pass your annual competencies, you need to notify the medical education department at the earliest possible opportunity, and if necessary, escalate to the foundation programme director about your troubles (C, B). Putting another date in the diary is not optimal as they have cancelled several times and this cannot be relied upon as a method of having a meeting (A). Unfortunately, a different consultant would unlikely be able to complete the form for you without the permission of the medical education department but is better than filling it in yourself which would be lying (D, E).

Question 181: ECABD

If you suspect a patient is being maltreated, you have a duty to act upon your suspicions. You should document what you saw and exactly what was said in the notes and escalate to the matron (E, C). In this case, it is not your role to apologise to the patient, therefore, filling in an incident report is more prudent (A, B). Doing nothing is unacceptable (D).

Question 182: BCDEA

In this case, a clinical error has been made. Therefore, you should refuse to sign the prescription and escalate immediately to your registrar or consultant (B, C). The ward sister should be informed after the patient has been clinically reviewed by a senior with an incident report filled out (D, E). Prescribing the fluid is dangerous and makes you liable if there is a consequence (A).

Question 207: DBAEC

When ordering investigations for a patient, you should know the background and be ready to answer clinical questions, particularly in the case of radiological investigations as the history helps the radiologist interpret scans. You should be honest by admitting you do not know much about the patient (D). The best source of information would be your registrar, but because they are busy, you should obtain the details and call the radiologist yourself (B). The next best option would be to look in the patient clerking (A). In an ideal scenario, the registrar would call the radiologist, but unfortunately, they are too busy in this case to do so (E). Inventing clinical symptoms is unprofessional (C).

Question 208: EBACD

With cuts to social care in the context of an ageing population, medically fit inpatients are increasingly having their discharge delayed by social problems. In this case, you should explore the patient's concerns (E). Next, notify the bed manager that it is unlikely she will be discharged (B). The patient will possibly need social service input (A). In this case, the patient is not disputing that they are medically fit to go home, therefore (C) ranks lower down. The final statement is a lie which makes it the worst option (D).

Question 209: BCDEA

Ultimately, it is the patient's decision how the final stage of their life is spent (B). However, it is also important to seek input from the family (C). The next appropriate option would be to arrange an MDT discussion involving the patient and their family (D). At that point, if the patient still wants to go to the hospice then the palliative care team can step in (E). Seeing how events unfold isn't appropriate as symptom control is still poor (A).

Question 210: BDECA

This question relates to communication skills. News such as this should really only be broken by a senior (B). You can, however, explore the patient's concerns about a potential diagnosis and their feelings about it (D). It would also be appropriate for you to suggest that further investigations may be needed before they can receive a diagnosis (E). (C) is a lie and thus inappropriate. Giving the patient false reassurance would be the worst possible option (A).

Question 211: CBAED

This relates to your ability to be pragmatic when it comes to patient safety. As the medications are not currently available, the best choice in the interim would be to prescribe an alternative, and seeking advice from the pharmacist is optimal (C). Ultimately, you should use the patient's own supply, so asking the family to provide that would be necessary (B). Prescribing a generic alternative drug is not ideal apart from in extreme circumstances or after specialist input as you will not have the experience to make that decision (A). It is not your choice to halt the medication or cross it out, but omitting until discharge is the better of the two remaining options (E, D).

Question 212: ACBED

The decision to approve your leave lies with your clinical supervisor (A). However, in this case, there is a valid reason for it not to be granted in that there will be no clinical cover (C). Notifying your educational supervisor in this case is likely to be irrelevant as is seeking legal advice due to the fact that this is not related to religious discrimination but to patient safety (B, E). Taking the day off sick risks patient safety and is the worst option (D).

Question 213: BECAD

In this scenario, you are supposed to be shadowing and should not be left to fend for yourself. You should notify the medical education department as soon as this occurs and seek advice from first the SHO as they would be more familiar with your tasks and furthermore are in your direct chain of command, and next the nursing staff (B, E, C). In terms of patient safety, it would not be safe for you to do the jobs as you may not be familiar with the systems and are liable to error. Therefore, counter-intuitively, (A) would still be better than (D).

Question 214: ECBAD

Your ability to consent depends on your seniority and whether you are able to convey the important benefits and complications of the procedure in a way that the patient can understand. As an FY1, you should never be in a position where you are consenting a patient. Therefore, you should explain that you cannot consent and ask the consultant who is supervising the line to do so (E, C). If the consultant cannot consent the patient for whatever reason, then the next best option is to ask one of the SHO's (B). Ultimately, having a consent form is necessary for the procedure so you doing one is better than not having one at all (A, D).

Question 215: ECBDA

Almost 8% of prescriptions have errors in them. In this scenario, you should call the on-call FY1 and notify them of the potential error (E). If they are unavailable, then the registrar is the next most appropriate (C). The next best alternative is to tell the nursing staff on the ward; however, direct doctor-to-doctor handover is always safer and thus the ideal to strive fort (B). The greatest risk to patient safety is to leave it until the morning, making this the worst choice (D, A).

Question 216: BDCEA

If a patient lacks capacity, it is wise to seek the approval of the next of kin for procedures (B). If not, then you should perform the procedure as it is in the patient's best interests (D). As the registrar is busy, it would not be appropriate to call them over the consultant (C, E). Because the patient likely requires the lumbar puncture, refusing to do it completely is the worst option (A).

Question 217: BEDAC

In this case, the least restrictive methods should be tried first including talking to the patient yourself and asking the next of kin for help (B, E). If this does not help, then you would have to section the patient under the mental health act (D). Physically restraining the patient can only be done if they are sectioned under the mental health act (A). It would be inappropriate to let the patient leave (C).

Question 218: EBACD

Such injuries are highly suspicious for being non-accidental. If this is suspected, you are required to take a full history and examination (E, B). You should also notify the designated clinician for child protection within your trust of your suspicions (A). As this is not a confirmed case of child abuse, informing the police would be premature, though the patient may later need to be separated from their parents (C). Discharging the patient puts the child at risk and is therefore completely inappropriate (D).

Question 219: DEACB
As you have attempted cannulation twice, and the nursing staff have also failed, then it is worthwhile asking your team – first your SHO, then your registrar regardless of whether or not they are asleep (D, E). The next best answer would be to ask for the help of the anaesthetist, but usually only after your team members have all tried (A). As the antibiotics are for meningitis, you cannot delay them until the morning, making this the worst answer (C, B).

Question 220: BEACD
In this case, you have a duty to protect the public from an infectious disease. If you cannot convince the patient to tell their partner, you should inform them that you will have to breach confidentiality and notify them yourself (B, E, A). You cannot withhold treatment from a patient in order to blackmail them into telling their partner, making this the worst option (C, D).

Question 221: DEBAC
In terms of organ donation, the specialist nurses coordinate family conversations and listing of organs so they are your first point of contact (D). Ultimately, the family's wishes will need to be respected regardless of whether the patient was on the organ donor register (E). Of the last three options, none are appropriate but respecting the patient's wishes would be the next best option (B). It would be better to dismiss the family (A) rather than informing the transplant team for public interest (C), the latter being wholly inappropriate and worse than just dismissing the family.

Question 222: BDF
In this case, the main issue is patient safety. You should initially discuss your concerns with the colleague involved (B) and state that they should not be taking time to study as you feel it is risking patient safety (F). You should also escalate your concerns to your registrar (D). Asking colleagues if they feel the same way would not make a difference to the need for you to take immediate action, as you already feel patient safety is being compromised.

Question 223: AEG
The two most sensible options in this scenario are to speak to your supervising consultant and educational supervisor as your professional development is being impaired (A, E). The third best option is close between organising teaching and organising a structured programme for the rotation (C, G). In the latter, you will be able to ensure you create a logbook which yourself and future trainees must accomplish to pass the rotation. This puts an onus on the consultants and supervisors to provide experience in clinical care such as clinical skills. This is why (G) is preferable to (C).

Question 224: BGH
As you speak to the nursing staff, the first thing to do would be to advise them not to give the antibiotic (G). The only way to get an accurate allergy history is usually from the patient or from their GP practice or old records (B). You should also amend the prescription if there is any doubt (H). Later on, you should consider escalating to the SHO on-call before the consultant and submitting an incident report which is why these are not in the top three responses.

Question 225: BEG
Errors can occur when transcribing results from one system to another. In this case, as you have noticed a potentially life-threatening abnormality, you should review the patient and treat them appropriately (E,G). In terms of clinical care, you should make your team aware of the error (B) and correct results as soon as possible.
You should apologise to the patient but only once they have been reviewed and are treated appropriately. This is the same for changing the details on your handover sheet and why these two options are not in the top three.

Question 226: DCEBA
Health service pressures dictate that finishing discharge summaries in a timely fashion is part of the job. In this case, the most pragmatic approach is to complete the discharge summary whilst handing over – multitasking is part of the job (D). If not, you should delay your handover in order to complete the discharge summary (C). Handing over to the registrar isn't usually appropriate unless it regards deteriorating patients, but at least the discharge summary will be done by someone who knows the patient (E). Handing over the discharge summary is the next option, but if the pharmacy is closed you may ultimately be better off doing it the next day yourself, however, this will delay the discharge further (B, A).

Question 227: BDEAC
The most appropriate thing to do is to notify the senior sister and then watch as the medication is given or do it yourself (B, D). Then you should notify your consultant of the clinical incident (E). It is worth emailing the night staff as there may have been a valid clinical reason as to why it could not be given, e.g. you could not obtain it from the pharmacy (A). An incident report would be mandatory in this scenario as well as an apology to the patient (C).

Question 228: CAEBD
This question relates to prioritisation. It is your team's responsibility that the bloods are taken in preparation for the next day. As the patient in A&E is unwell, the best thing to do would be to handover to the night team to do the bloods (C). The next best solution would be to ask the nursing staff (A). As your current patient is unwell, it would be inappropriate to ask the registrar to leave this patient to carry out a task that could easily be delegated to someone else(E). Of the last two options, putting the bloods out for the next day risks delay which may mean postponement of the operation, therefore, that is the worst answer (B, D).

Question 229: BCG
In this case, the patient needs antibiotics urgently for a potentially life-threatening infection. The best option would be to check if your SHO or registrar knows what antibiotics to give and the dose and duration as this won't impede the ward round (C). If not, you should prescribe the drug only once you know what to give and how much. These could be determined from the hospital formulary or the BNF (G, B). A fellow FY1 would likely not have the experience to know what to give, and you should not just prescribe an antibiotic as it may not be appropriate for that indication.

Question 230: BDH
In this case, it states that news has been given to the patient but it does not specifically mention lung cancer. Therefore, you should establish a baseline as to what they currently understand (D). You should be honest stating that you are unlikely to have the knowledge to answer their questions and seek senior advice (B, H). It is not the nursing staff's responsibility to contact your seniors to break the news; that lies with a member of your team. If none of the above methods work, the next step would be that they ask the next day (A).

Question 231: ABD
If a family member wishes to stay in the room during resuscitation they usually should be allowed, unless they are becoming obstructive to resuscitation attempts – which in this scenario it doesn't appear they are. You should check on them during the attempt as the chaotic atmosphere may be too much and they can feel trapped once they decide to stay (A). If they are there, it is best that they are in a corner to reduce any impact they are having on the clinical team (B). It is also nice to designate someone to be with them to explain what is happening as it can be a frightening experience (D). In this case, you do not know if resuscitation will be successful as you have just arrived. Option (G) is suboptimal; just because he isn't bothering you doesn't mean the son isn't bothering others.

Question 232: BEG
This is an extremely common occurrence. The first thing should be to apologise to the patient, it is no fault of their own that the notes are unavailable (G). It would be wise to attempt to contact the GP surgery to try and get some background (E). In any case, even if you do not have the medical history then you should still take a history and examine the patient (B). Making another appointment to come back can be done but is a use of additional resources, therefore, it is less optimal than seeing how much you can do at the time in the clinic. You should fill in an incident report but at a later stage. You should not list the patient for surgery without a full medical history as they may need further medical input for optimisation before being considered.

Question 233: AEG
After a traumatic experience, there can be an emotional reaction from anyone involved. This question looks at the way you react and treat other colleagues with compassion. The most appropriate thing to do in this case would be to notify the facilitators (E). The team should allow her some time and space to cry (G). The next best option would be to speak to her yourself after the session, though not immediately, as this gives her space and time to think (A). It is best you do this (rather than her nursing colleagues) as you were there in the situation with her and have the same emotions. Giving her a hug is inappropriate and reporting her via an incident form is overkill given that no actual patients have to come to harm and this is a training session.

Question 234: CDF
This is a common occurrence as patients tend not to bring medications to hospital when they come acutely. The best answers for this scenario are the ones that will provide the most up-to-date information surrounding their drug history. This is therefore the next of kin, ambulance sheet, and GP records (C, D, F). Previous discharge summaries would be a close fourth, but may be outdated.

Question 235: BDH
Needlestick and blood splash injuries have protocols that should be followed when they do occur. Irrigation is the first and most immediate treatment (D). You should then leave to go to accident and emergency for your bloods to be taken (B). Never ask others in the vicinity to take them (G). Bloods should be taken from the patient but ideally after they have consented, not intra-operatively (H).

Question 236: CDH
In this scenario, it is your responsibility to ensure that the whole shift is covered until the end. Calling in sick is unprofessional and leaving early and leaving the team one member down for two hours risks patient safety. The best option is to swap the entire shift (C). If that is not possible, then you should do the shift to completion (D). The third best option would be to ask the night FY1 to come in early as you would be doing them a favour in return so it can be mutually beneficial (H). A close fourth would be to ask the FY1 who is on the next day to do the last two hours (B) – but it is unfair to make them add an extra two hours to their shift.

Question 237: BEG
In this case, you feel patient safety has the potential to be compromised so you have a duty to act. You should first speak to the SHO and address your concerns directly to see if there is any way you might be able to resolve them (B). If not, you need to escalate to your consultant registrar so they are aware of the situation (G, E). If problems are severe, the next stage would be notifying the service manager. Your educational supervisor wouldn't really have any input in this scenario.

Question 238: BFG
This is a tough situation as it puts ethical principles up against NHS rationing of resources. In this case, the answers would likely be subjective and based on the examiner's feelings as a cohort – there may not even be agreement amongst themselves. We collectively felt as medical practitioners that the best two options would be to treat the patient (B, F). The next best option would be to ask for advice from the team that deal with international patients and private healthcare (G). Asking the consultant to see the patient won't add anything at this stage, nor would discussing this with the nurse in charge.

Question 239: BDG
In this case, the consent will not be valid unless the patient fully understands the consequences and you are sure that the opinion is given without undue external pressure. Therefore, you should tell the wife that unless she translates word for word, the consent would not be valid and you will not be able to perform the procedure (B). If that does not work, the next best option, seeing as this would be an elective procedure, would be to rearrange the appointment with a formal translator (D). As the wife is what is limiting the consent, asking her to leave the room and using an online tool would be preferable as the next option, compared to asking a colleague to translate with her still present (G). Listing the patient is ethically inappropriate when there are concerns about the validity of his consent.

Question 240: BEF
Good Medical Practice states that you should avoid treating friends and relatives whenever possible. The most appropriate option would be to notify the registrar and ask the SHO to see the patient (B, F). If you do see the patient, you should consent them to ensure they are happy with you being involved in their care (E). All the other options result in incomplete or no clinical assessment of the patient which compromises patient safety.

Question 241: BCE

As the patient is sitting upright and verbalising, there is no immediate rush to see the patient. Preparation is essential. Asking the nursing staff to do the observations is prudent whilst you are on the way to see the patient (B). You should look through the notes to get a background summary of the patient then take a history (E, C). In other scenarios, doing an ABCDE assessment first would be appropriate, especially if the patient were unwell.

Question 242: ADE

When patients have similar names, it is the responsibility of all the staff to ensure that they are aware and are extra careful in order to avoid clinical errors. In this case, you should immediately notify the nurse in charge of what has occurred (A). You should then apologise to the patient who was inappropriately exposed to radiation (E). Next, you should ensure the correct patient has the scan booked (D). Later, you should notify your consultant of the error and incident report it. You could also consider apologising to the patient awaiting the scan, notifying them of what happened.

Question 243: CDF

If you are unwell, particularly with nausea and vomiting, you are putting patients at risk of illness such as norovirus. Therefore, you should notify medical staff and go home (C). Ensure your team and consultant are aware of the situation (D). Leaving without notifying anyone is bad practice (F), but is better for patient safety than continuing and taking anti-sickness medication.

Question 244: BEG

Whilst the question mentions that patient safety may be compromised as a result of Tom's action, the key here is that you have not witnessed this. Hence, your role in mediating this situation is more supportive rather than active. Therefore, the best option is to get Jenny to speak to Tom directly (B) as this allows them to have a frank and open discussion. If this fails then Jenny should speak to a senior colleague (registrar/consultant) to voice her concerns (E) as this is the proper protocol for escalation. Additionally, Jenny should seek the opinion of other members of the medical team to see if her views are echoed by them (G) – she needs to be sure that Tom is putting patient safety at risk by getting more information before she escalates the issue. Explaining that you haven't noticed Tom acting this way (A) is not idea as it doesn't address Jenny's concerns and potentially makes her feel isolated. Speaking to Tom directly yourself (C), to the other FY1s (F) or informing a senior colleague (D) is not correct as it would be unfair to accuse him based on Jenny's observations. Emailing the team consultant (H) is too heavy handed given the lack of information in the question – this scenario requires a more delicate approach.

Question 245: ABG

In this case, the safety of yourself, the staff, and patients is paramount. Therefore, security should be involved as early as possible (A). Attempt to de-escalate the situation yourself verbally if possible and if it is safe to do so (B). However, you should make it clear that this behaviour is not acceptable (G). It is difficult to say if the behaviour is due to a head injury or alcohol. Initially, you should focus on the aggressive patient and later you can apologise to other patients and check they are okay. If none of your measures are working, you will need to move other patients away and isolate the threat.

Question 246: BEG

This relates to a combination of communication and patient safety. Microbiology have decided to start a certain antibiotic deliberately, and therefore, you should challenge your consultant's reasoning after explaining what microbiology explained the day before (E, B). You should not change the antibiotics without consulting the microbiology team (G). Ultimately, this is a clinical decision, although pharmacists can be a useful adjunct. It isn't up to the patient to decide what antibiotics they receive.

Question 247: BCG

This relates to patient safety, professional relationships and keeping things in confidence. Although there doesn't seem to be a risk to patient safety at the moment, a doctor who does not like reviewing patients could jeopardise this. You should initially have a confidential meeting with Ashwin and explore his fears (B). However, you should encourage him to speak to his clinical supervisor and occupational health regarding the issue to see if they can provide additional support during his training and minimise risk to patients (C, G). An educational supervisor may become involved at a later date. You should only speak to your supervisor if Ashwin refuses. Notifying colleagues and nursing staff breaches Ashwin's confidentiality and there is no need for them to know at this stage.

Question 248: BDH

As there is a life-threatening medical problem here, you should immediately perform an ABCDE assessment and begin appropriate treatment (B, D). In cases of potential anaphylaxis, you should escalate it immediately (H). All the other options are valid responses but should be done later, once the patient has been stabilised.

Question 249: CEF

Mental health problems are common in the medical profession due to the physical and emotional demands of the job. In this instance, making an appointment to see your GP is the best place to start (C). If you think your work is being affected, then you have a duty to notify your clinical supervisor to protect patient safety (E). You should also seek advice from occupational health about whether a period of leave would be beneficial (F). Seeking advice from colleagues is a good idea, but it will, making it the next best option but not in the top three. You should not start medication without input from a GP.

Question 250: AEBCD

(A) is the best answer. You have correctly prioritised the more unwell patient, resisted the temptation to prescribe without assessing the patient, but also given the nurse a timeframe and alternative techniques whilst she waits. Bleeping your registrar isn't ideal when you could manage both patients consecutively but at least both patients will be fully assessed €. Prescribing a drug without assessing the patient is dangerous as a rule. The patient may be agitated because he's in urinary retention, in pain, delirious from sepsis etc., but prescribing a sedative is better than doing nothing at all for this patient (B, C). (D) is the worst option as this patient is deteriorating and shouldn't be left without a plan in place.

Question 251: CDABE

(C) is most appropriate as it flags the mistake early in the day so it can be rectified with least disruption. Asking a friend on another specialty isn't ideal as he will have his own responsibilities and time pressures, but if he has the time and is willing to do it for you, it does solve the issue efficiently (D). You are off and should not return to the hospital for a problem that could be solved by a phone call, however, bleeding the patient yourself is better than the patient not being bled at all until 7PM when the drug is due (A). Lying about the urgency of a blood test is a poor option (B) as this jeopardises the safety of other patients by slowing down the list of urgent blood tests with non-urgent ones. However, doing nothing is the worst option overall (E).

Question 252: BDEAC

Signing the register for him is dishonest, hence (A) ranks poorly. Offering to go to a meeting with the foundation programme lead with him for moral support is a good answer (E), however it ranks poorly because you have dishonestly signed the register. It is best he speaks directly with the head of the foundation programme himself (B), but failing that, (D) serves the same purpose. (C) is the worst of all options as it involves directly lying to him *and* dissuades him from contacting the head of the foundation programme because he believes he's getting away with it.

Question 253: ECBAD

This one is self-explanatory. (E) is the most appropriate and practical response, followed by (C). It is deceitful to do these forms without him having witnessed you perform the procedures. However, it is more dishonest to have a difficult one signed off rather than the ones that you could honestly say you are proficient at (B, A). Reporting him to the deanery would risk his career and is a step too far, especially as he was only offering to help you (D).

Question 254: CEBDA

You must alert the ward that you will be late and offer an alternative doctor to contact in the event a patient becomes acutely unwell (C).). Giving the bleep number of a fellow FY1 who is on the scene is more appropriate than immediately escalating something potentially trivial to the consultant who is busy in a meeting (E). If your fellow FY1 is unable to manage the problem, they know how to escalate appropriately. Offering your mobile number when you are not onsite and are currently driving is unhelpful as you cannot assess the patient over the phone (B). Contacting your consultant without telling the ward (D) is irritating as the consultant will then have to let the ward know who to contact in the event of needing a doctor. Not even mentioning the fact that you will be late and giving alternative contacts is the worst option (A).

Question 255: DBACE

The most appropriate answers involve discussing it with your colleague. Aiming to keep things fair and improve your learning by alternating who goes to theatre is the best option (D) followed by ensuring that your colleague doesn't leave you with an unfair workload in order to improve his career prospects (B). Discussing the issue with the operating surgeon (A) is not ideal as you should try to resolve the situation with your colleague before escalating it. Raising the issue to a senior level prematurely has the potential to impact your working relationship. Accepting the problem (C) is not fair on you as your learning suffers and you shouldn't be doing all the ward work alone. However, it is preferable to (E) which is too extreme at this stage, especially as you have not even attempted to discuss it with your colleague first!

Question 256: ECDAB

The most appropriate answers involve learning the skills you are weak at in a safe environment. The best option is to book a slot at the clinical skills lab (E) as this allows you to practice the procedure without the risk of harming patients. This is preferable to practicing on real patients given that you've never seen the procedure done. The next best option is to teach each other the skills (C). Attempting to do catheters on your own having not seen it done before is not ideal (D) and puts patients at risk of UTIs – you should ideally practice on a model or with a supervisor first. However, you are attempting to preserve patient safety and comfort by only having one attempt which is much preferable to option (B). Option (A) is only slightly better than (B) as although you won't be causing patients' harm, you will never learn to catheterise.

Question 257: BCDEA

(B) is most appropriate as it ensures patient safety whilst trying to avoid similar situations arising again. (C) isn't perfect as this is not a one-off, impacting on your personal life, and it is likely that you will be tired as it states you have worked until 8PM all week. Leaving the bleep with the SHO ensures (D) someone is present to answer the bleep, but the SHO will have their own responsibilities and patients to cover. However, they are preferable to the remaining options. Calling your educational supervisor at 8PM on a Friday isn't likely to be fruitful (E). Leaving a bleep uncovered and a list of jobs on the computer that she may not find (A) risks patient safety- you don't know if she will turn up at all!

Question 258: CDEAB

If someone smells strongly of alcohol, it is likely they have consumed alcohol very recently and thus are a potential risk to patients. You are never expected to tackle your consultant alone regarding such a difficult issues. Therefore, you should speak to your registrar immediately (C) so that they can approach the consultant and involve other team members as necessary. The next best option is to call your educational supervisor (D) as they will be a consultant and thus able to approach the surgeon on an equal footing. However, they are unlikely to be available straight away because they will be on a different team/hospital and hence it's better to contact the registrar to get immediate help. Confronting the surgeon directly (E) addresses the issue but is likely to be inflammatory and your concerns might not be taken seriously. This is still preferable to ignoring the issue (A) as that risks patient safety. Being complicit in this scenario by helping the surgeon mask his breathe (B) is grossly inappropriate.

Question 269: CDE

Confidentiality and respectful treatment of all patients is an essential hallmark of good medical care. Not only is it disrespectful and unprofessional to publicly judge patients, it is also a potential breach of confidentiality, depending on the issues discussed. This, in turn, is a significant breach of protocol with associated consequences. By informing the clinic manager, you ensure that appropriate steps are being taken to prevent this issue from reoccurring (C). The same applies to having a private word with the person in question. This will make her error clear to her (E). Apologising to the patient present will ensure that the professional relationship in the workplace is maintained and not threatened by the behaviour of the individual (D).

Question 270: BFH

The patient's ability to consent requires assessment under consideration of Gillick competence. This is something that is best done at the GP's practice since the patient is in hospital for a completely unrelated issue. Requesting the OCP from her GP ensures that appropriate monitoring is possible. The GP is also more likely to know the girl better than you do, so will be able to make an informed judgement not only of her competence under Gillick, but also of her personal situation with regards to her unprotected sex (B, F). Providing the patient with information, however, does not require any monitoring, nor does it require a close knowledge of the patient's personal background, and is therefore always advisable (H).

Question 271: AGH

The underlying issue here is prescription safety. Since both, Bumetanide and Furosemide are loop diuretics, they should not be co-administered unless there is exceptionally good reason to do so otherwise they might lead to electrolyte abnormalities and drug interactions. You need to ascertain whether this prescription was done in error or was intentional. The best way to do this is to either speak to your colleague directly (A), review the medical notes to see if they've mentioned their rationale for adding Bumetanide (G) or speak to a senior doctor for a second opinion (H). The key thing here is that the patient has not actually had Bumetanide so has not come to any harm. Hence, informing them (D) and completing an incident form (B) is not necessary. Rewriting the drug chart without proper consultation (E and F) is not advisable.

Question 272: BDE

There are several important considerations at play in this question. Firstly, your own protection. By documenting your treatment plan and the conversation you had with the registrar, you ensure that any outcome cannot impact you negatively. Discussing the issue with the registrar in private will give you the opportunity to provide justification for your diagnosis and will also make it easier for the registrar to change his mind and treat the leg as compartment syndrome (D, E). If all these steps prove unsuccessful, escalating the issue to the orthopaedic consultant will provide a way to solve the problem through hierarchical decision making (B).

Question 273: CGH
The consideration at the core of this issue is patient safety. Making a mistake is always possible, but it is the approach to the consequences that makes the difference. By filling in the incidence form and raising the issue with the nurse and ward sister, you ensure that all appropriate steps are taken in response to the mistake (G). Contacting the family is essential as any adverse effects need to be put into context and addressed as soon as possible in order to optimise the outcome (C). Asking for senior help is always a safe bet (H).. As an FY1, you are still at the beginning of your training and nobody expects you to be flawless. Problems only arise if you try to hide your mistakes.

Question 274: AEF
Providing the patient with all the necessary information is vital in this case. Clearly, it would be preferable for the patient to complete the tests in order to guide further management, but you cannot force the patient to accept any treatment (E). If he chooses to ignore your advice and self-discharge, it is advisable to document the conversation. Often, aggression and frustration from the patient is a result of poor communication between the patient and clinician. By taking the time to listen to the patient's concerns, you can ensure an appropriate and responsible approach to their worries. This, in turn, makes them more likely to listen to you (A, F).

Question 275: ABD
Any person with capacity is entitled to make any decision about the treatment they desire. Disagreeing with a decision does not mean that we can ignore the patient's view. If the patient is of capacity, it is his right to refuse the treatment (A, D). Exploring his motivation in this case is essential to gain an understanding of his actions (B). Issues of death and end-of-life care are difficult but necessary topics to discuss, especially if the patient brings it up. Finally, it is important to document the conversation in order to ensure that there is no ambiguity surrounding the context in which the decision is made.

Question 276: ACE
Considering that the patient may not have capacity, leaving the ward could pose a significant risk to himself and others. Stopping him from leaving is therefore in his best interest and thus getting the patient back to the ward should be your first priority (A). Considering that he has assaulted a nurse, it seems wise to keep a distance and contact security who are trained to manage such situations (C). It is not advisable to put yourself in harm's way, which is why trying to have a conversation from a safe distance is an appropriate decision. Invasive methods such as sedation or physical violence are completely inappropriate and the same applies to ignoring the situation.

Question 277: BEG
The key consideration in this question is teamwork and appropriateness. The registrar's comments are not appropriate in any situation. They do not contribute to a healthy and efficient working environment. Hence, the issue should be raised with the registrar, and other team members (B, E). If this is an isolated incident, there is no reason to escalate the issue further, but if it recurs, the consultant should be informed (F). Ignoring the incident is also inappropriate as it does not contribute to a healthy working environment.

Question 278: CGH
Medicine is a career with a lot of pressure, thus it is common for health professionals to need support. Discussing the colleague's feelings with her can provide her with help and a feeling of support that can be very beneficial in her situation (C). Offering to support her with the consultant in question may allow her to have this important conversation as she will feel less alone. The same general principle applies for you encouraging her to have a conversation with her FY2 (H). Whilst all the other options seem to tackle parts of the problem, these three choices are the most reasonable and readily feasible.

Question 279: ADF
The core consideration here is patient safety. If a doctor is not obtainable when he is needed, he is not doing his job and is putting patients at risk. This is an issue that needs to be dealt with urgently. By involving the responsible consultant, the problem is raised in an official capacity, enabling appropriate steps to be taken to avoid it from happening again (A). Arranging a meeting with the ST3 is another reasonable course of action as this will give him the benefit of the doubt and a chance to explain himself (D). The critical incident form is another way in which an official inquiry into the issue can be started (F). Ultimately, any step that reinstates patient safety is a good solution to this problem. Harsher steps such as reporting the doctor to the GMC are options that need to be considered more carefully. Ignoring the problem is also a poor choice as this will mean that patients continue to be put at risk by the doctor's behaviour.

Question 280: BAEDC
This is actually not an uncommon situation. This question tests your ability to recognise your own limits and to get help appropriately. Given that the patient has several acute and chronic problems that have not been investigated, the best option is for a medical senior to review them in person (B), followed by on the phone (A). Speaking to another orthopaedic registrar is the next best option as they are likely to have more experience than you of medical management and may give you more sensible advice than your own registrar (E). Assessing the patient to the best of your ability (D) is not ideal given that this patient would require multiple investigations and conflicting treatments that are best managed by a senior. Even worse is to ignore these issues altogether and just follow the registrar's plan (C)

Question 281: BACDE
This is a dangerous situation as although she currently does not appear drunk; there is a risk that she might become more intoxicated over the next few hours (especially if she continues drinking). Hence, it's paramount that you protect patient safety by informing your seniors (B) so that they can put disciplinary measures into place as well as arrange appropriate junior doctor cover in her absence.

The next best option is to protect patient safety by offering to cover her shift. It's better to be supportive (A) as there might be pastoral reasons for her drinking (difficult job, divorce, financial hardship etc). Offering to cover her shift alone does not prevent the issue from happening again (C). Informing her educational supervisor if the issue recurs is sensible (D) but this option lacks any acute response which is necessary in this situation. Ignoring the situation entirely is the worst option as it risks patient safety (E).

Question 282: CEABD
The rationale in this question is to follow the procedure that is the most defensible in a court of law, as well as with the individual opinion. Being true to yourself and to trust your instincts is always important (C). Similarly, it is important to realise the superior clinical experience of the consultant (E) and the registrar (A), that exceeds yours at this point of your training. Consulting the coroner's office would be advisable if the death is unexplainable or unexpected, in which case, wrongdoing can be suspected (B). Refusing to complete the death certificate is a poor choice assuming that there is no indication of a wrongful death as this will leave the family of the deceased in unnecessary distress. Considering their already highly emotional situation, it would not be appropriate to cause them further distress by refusing to fill in the certificate (D).

Question 283: BACED
The underlying issue in this question is prescription safety and control. By refusing to prescribe antibiotics to your wife and asking her to register with a GP, you avoid any problems from a legal perspective (B). Although the GMC advises to avoid prescribing for friends and family, a single private prescription of antibiotics (that are not controlled drugs like opiates) is unlikely to be viewed too unfavourably here (A). It is better to prescribe the medication privately rather than through the hospital (C) as the latter implies that you are her responsible clinician and would also cost the hospital money (as the drugs would be billed to the hospital). Asking a colleague to prescribe on your behalf for your wife puts them in a tricky position as they are also unlikely to want to take responsibility as her clinician (E). Prescribing in another person's name is the worst option – not only is it illegal, the prescription will also get linked to the other patient's medical records (D).

Question 284: CEBDA
The underlying issue here is confidentiality. In theory, you are not allowed to give out any information regarding a patient to a third person without their explicit consent. In addition, since the friend's father was admitted to a different department, you are not a part of his care and are therefore not entitled to access the information related to his care, even though you are theoretically able to. In practice, there is somewhat of a grey area surrounding this issue. For this reason, the best course of action, working under the assumption that your friend's father does not object to your friend knowing about his illness, is to get written permission for your enquiry (C). If this cannot be achieved, rejection is the safest course of action (E). Providing your friend with the required information should then be raised with the treating team in order to find the reason for the hospital's rejection of information sharing (B). By asking the friend's father to get in touch with her, all issues surrounding confidentiality are avoided (D). Involving another third party (your consultant) is the worst course of action as it would be a further breach of confidentiality (A).

Question 285: ADBCE

Honesty is always the best course of action. If you feel that you are not able to fulfil your work duties as well as the two audits with sufficient quality, being honest about this is the best thing to do. It makes clear that you are a responsible clinician and are aware of your limitations. By offering to find somebody else to do the project, you prove yourself helpful and interested rather than lazy (A). Accepting the audit on top of your already existing work can be a challenging decision, but if you feel that you can do an appropriately good job by using your half days for the additional audit, you can accept in order to advance your academic skills (D). Flatly refusing can be misunderstood and can impair your professional perception by the consultant (B). Dishonest behaviour does not help anybody, and by either banking on the consultant forgetting about the project (C) or by deliberately avoiding doing the work and shifting it to your successor (E), you undermine your own credibility for making these two choices, therefore, they are the least appropriate.

Question 286: ACBDE

In general, there is no reason for you not to go and cannulate the patient just because he is in the private wing of the hospital. The best option is assess the urgency of the transfusion and cannulate if necessary (A) – even if it's not your direct responsibility as you must not knowingly cause harm to patients (even if they aren't under your care!). Double checking with the duty manager regarding the appropriateness of you cannulating the patient is also a good option as this will ensure that you are not acting out of position and putting yourself in a potentially incriminating position (C). In an ideal world, the private ward should have someone who can cannulate (B) however telling the receptionist that is unlikely to lead to a change in their policy and merely creates bad-will.

Leaving an invoice for the cannula is not a good idea as it is not your patient, and the mere fact that they are on the private ward does not entitle you to charge them for your service (D). However, that is still better than flat out refusing to cannulate (E) regardless of the clinical context is not advisable as if the patient comes to harm, you could still find yourself in a difficult legal position.

Question 287: ABECD

This question addresses the general issue of confidentiality and the degree of information sharing that is appropriate. In general, there is specific legislation governing this situation, especially situations when confidentiality must be broken and when it can be to a limited extent. In this case, it is reasonable to assume that laws such as the Terrorism Act do not apply. In general, you do not have to share any information with the police, unless there is a risk for the general health or specific laws apply to the individual situation (A). When in doubt, consulting with a superior for guidance is always a smart decision as it moves the responsibility for the situation from you to somebody else who has more experience (B). In the event that you choose to share information, sharing the least amount of information possible is also a solution (E). As mentioned above, there are instances when confidential information has to be or can be released (C). (D) is the least appropriate solution as it is an attempt to avoid responsibility in this situation which is not a good demonstration of character.

Question 288: BCDEA

The key issue here is that airway management is the most important factor in resuscitation. Whilst an anaesthetist normally manages the airway, the best response here is to directly address the issue and clarify why no one is managing the airway (B). Asking for an anaesthetist (C) is the next best option as they might be present and busy with other tasks or they may well be on their way. It is worse than option B as its more long winded approach and doesn't directly address the main issue.

By supporting with chest compressions (D), you can provide a positive influence to the situation and potentially free up other people to deal with the patient's airway. Inaction is a poor choice, as this does not contribute to changing the situation at hand (E). In an arrest situation, it is important to maintain order which is why jumping in without instruction is the least appropriate choice for this scenario (A) - not to mention that you are unlikely to be equipped to deal with airway management in your first week as a doctor!

Question 289: BAECD

There are two main considerations at play in this scenario. On one hand, this is patient safety that needs to be maintained at all times, and on the other hand, you must act within the limits of your competence. If you execute a procedure you do not feel comfortable executing by yourself, you leave yourself in a vulnerable position and open to litigation should something go wrong. By declining to place the catheter, you ensure that both aspects are taken into account (B). If there is somebody with experience in this procedure that can assist and supervise you with the task, doing the procedure carries less risk and can be a good learning experience (A). If there is no supervision available and you still choose to undertake the procedure, appropriate documentation is vital as this will protect you to some degree (E). The two remaining points are equally as inappropriate because they either ignore the patient's needs (C) or delay the task at hand (D).

Question 290: CABED

The essential part here is that she needs to understand the consequences and dangers of her actions - this is only possible if you provide the information in an accessible way and if she has the capacity to make the decision (A). Since the patient is competent, there is no legal basis for keeping her in the hospital against her wishes, as long as you provide her with all the information associated with the risks associated with leaving the hospital (C). Advising her to seek help from her GP if the cellulitis worsens is necessary, but not sufficient by itself. Therefore, it presents a suboptimal option, especially since the patient requires IV antibiotics which are difficult to administer in the community (B). As the patient is competent, there are no legal grounds to hold her against her will (E). The least appropriate solution here is to get the patient's boyfriend involved as this would mean to exert undue pressure on her decision making which, in itself, is unacceptable (D).

Question 291: BACDE

This is a common clinical scenario and the most pragmatic solution is also the best one here – ie asking for a staff member who speaks the same language (B). This is likely to be much quicker and easier to arrange than a professional interpreter (A) which is the next best option. Asking the child to interpret (C) is not ideal given their age and the fact that the parent may not wish to disclose some information to their child or cause them any undue worry. Since the patient has come to A & E, there is clearly something urgent that they wish to address so asking them to go to their GP (D) is not appropriate however, this is still better than refusing to see the patient altogether (E) which risks patient safety.

Question 299: ACEBD
Communication here is the key in order to maintain a productive and efficient work environment. Giving the colleague the opportunity to explain himself in an uncharged and non-judgemental environment will ensure that the conversation can be productive (A). By discussing the issue with the colleague's educational supervisor, the issue will be raised in a professional environment (C). Whilst ignoring the issue here could be understandable and also acceptable, it does not contribute to the resolution of the unfavourable situation which makes it less appropriate (E). Sharing the situation with others is inappropriate as it makes the colleague look bad and puts him in an embarrassing situation that can be easily avoided (B). The same applies for demanding a public explanation. This form of public humiliation is unacceptable and is unlikely to result in favourable outcomes (D).

Question 300: BCDEA
Remember that patients are your greatest priority. If your patients aren't being reviewed by a senior doctor, they are getting poor care, and therefore, their safety could be potentially compromised. Thus, your aim should be to ensure that there are weekly senior ward rounds without damaging your professional relationship. Hence, (B) is the best decision as it is minimally confrontational yet firm. (C) is also a good idea as your supervisor may be able to speak to your consultant. However, it is best to approach them after you have at least raised the issue with your consultant first. (D) is a bit too extreme and will damage your relationship, although it does protect patient safety. (E) is not a very practical solution as you're unlikely to be as helpful given your experience and it does not resolve the core issue (your consultant's priorities being in the wrong place). (A) is the worst choice as you are enabling poor patient care.

FINAL ADVICE

Arrive well rested, well fed, and well hydrated

The SJT is an intensive test, so make sure you're ready for it. You'll have to sit this at a fixed time so get a good night's sleep before the exam (there is little point cramming) and don't miss breakfast. If you're taking water into the exam, then make sure you've been to the toilet before in order to avoid leaving during the exam. Make sure you're well rested and fed in order to be at your best!

Move On

If you're struggling, answer the question anyway and move on. Every question has equal weighting and there is no negative marking. In the time it takes to answer one hard question, you could gain three times the marks by answering the easier ones. Be smart to score points.

Complex Questions

- If there are several people mentioned in the scenario, make sure you are answering about the correct person.
- Think of what you 'should' do rather than what you necessarily would do.
- Always think of patient safety and acting in the patient's best interests.

Afterword

Remember that the route to a high score is your approach and practice. Don't fall into the trap that "*you can't prepare for the SJT*'– this could not be further from the truth. With knowledge of the test, some useful score-boosting-strategies, and plenty of practice, you can dramatically raise your score.

Work hard, never give up and do yourself justice. Good luck!

Acknowledgements

Many thanks to the doctors and tutors who took the time to contribute questions for this publication. Special thanks to *Aayushi* for her innovative artwork.

YOUR FREE BOOK

Thanks for purchasing this Ultimate Book. Readers like you have the power to make or break a book – hopefully you found this one useful and informative. *The Oxbridge Medical Society* would love to hear about your experiences with this book. As thanks for your time we'll send you another ebook from our Ultimate Guide series absolutely FREE!

How to Redeem Your Free Ebook

1) Find the book you have on your Amazon purchase history or your email receipt to help find the book on Amazon.

2) On the product page at the Customer Reviews area, click 'Write a customer review'. Write your review and post it! Copy the review page or take a screen shot of the review you have left.

3) Head over to **https://www.uniadmissions.co.uk/oxbridge-free-book/** and select your chosen free ebook!

Your ebook will then be emailed to you – it's as simple as that!

WWW.EXAMS.NINJA/FPAS-SJT/

Printed and bound by CPI Group (UK) Ltd, Croydon, CR0 4YY
02/11/2026
02243550-0001